Essentials
of Clinical
Neurophysiology

Essentials of Clinical Neurophysiology

Karl E. Misulis, M.D., Ph.D.

Assistant Clinical Professor of Neurology
Vanderbilt University
Nashville, Tennessee

Neurologist
Semmes-Murphey Clinic
Jackson, Tennessee

Butterworth–Heinemann
Boston   London   Oxford   Singapore   Sydney   Toronto   Wellington

Every effort has been made to ensure that the drug dosage schedules within this text are accurate and conform to standards accepted at time of publication. However, as treatment recommendations vary in the light of continuing research and clinical experience, the reader is advised to verify drug dosage schedules herein with information found on product information sheets. This is especially true in cases of new or infrequently used drugs.

Recognizing the importance of preserving what has been written, it is the policy of Butterworth–Heinemann to have the books it publishes printed on acid-free paper, and we exert our best efforts to that end.

Part I is derived in part from Misulis, K. E. Basic electronics for clinical neurophysiology. *Journal of Clinical Neurophysiology* 6 (1989): 41–74, and is used with permission of the publisher.

Library of Congress Cataloging-in-Publication Data

Misulis, Karl E.
    Essentials of clinical neurophysiology / Karl E. Misulis.
        p.   cm.
    Includes bibliographical references and index.
    ISBN 0-7506-9305-3 (hardcover)
    1. Electroencephalography.   2. Electromyography.   3. Evoked potentials (Electrophysiology)   4. Neurophysiology.   5. Neural conduction.   I. Title.
    [DNLM: 1. Electroencephalography—methods.   2. Electromyography—methods.   3. Evoked Potentials—physiology.   4. Neural Conduction—physiology.   5. Neurophysiology—methods.   WL 102 M6784e]
    RC386.6.E43M57   1993
    616.8'047547—dc20
    DNLM/DLC
    for Library of Congress   92–49457
                                                                              CIP

British Library Cataloguing-in-Publication Data

A catalogue record for this book is available from the British Library.

Butterworth–Heinemann
80 Montvale Avenue
Stoneham, MA 02180

10 9 8 7 6 5 4 3 2 1

Printed in the United States of America

To my parents, Edward and Ruth Misulis

□ □ □
□ □ □
□ □ □

Contents

□ □ □
□ □ □
□ □ □

Preface

Clinical neurophysiology encompasses most common neurodiagnostic techniques, including electroencephalography, electromyography with nerve conductions, evoked potentials, and polysomnography. This field has blossomed in the past ten years with increasing demand for many of these studies. Like all tests, the clinical utility is limited by the experience and training of the interpreter.

This book presents the essentials of clinical neurophysiology. It is intended for people new to neurodiagnostics and for those who want to learn more about selected neurodiagnostic techniques. The goal of this book is to provide the reader with a single source to guide competent performance and interpretation of these tests. This is not meant to be a substitute for comprehensive texts, but rather a complement, tying together the theories and practice of electrophysiology.

The first section reviews basic electronics and describes the function of neurodiagnostic equipment. Subsequent sections describe the methods and interpretation of electroencephalography, electromyography, evoked potentials, and polysomnography. A glossary and bibliography are presented at the end.

The typical drawback to a single-authored text is reading only one view. Most of the theories and recommendations are fairly standard, however. There should be little controversy about performance of the studies. In interpretation, I tend to be conservative in both my practice and writing. There is still considerable room for individual expertise and experience, giving opinions based on "close calls." For help with these interpretations, the reader should consult comprehensive texts and atlases in addition to this book.

Acknowledgments

I would like to acknowledge the enormous help of Dr. Gerald Fenichel for review of the manuscript. I also would like to express appreciation to Barbara Page and Laura Rushing for years of superb secretarial support.

The following were instrumental in advice, review of the manuscript, and screening tracings: Drs. Bassell Abou-Khalil, Toufic Fakhoury, Anthony Kilroy, Edwin Peguero, and Christa Stoscheck.

This book would have been impossible without the excellent work of the technicians: Teri Blunkall, Charlie Carroll, Jan "Typo" Johnson, Carolyn Kreppel, Karen Newman, Sue "Artifact" Olson, Sheryl Richardson, Kathy Roe, and Connie Webb.

Last but not least, I appreciate the patience of my wife, Dr. Christa Stoscheck, for putting up with me during the completion of this project.

□ □ □
□ □ □
□ □ □

List of Abbreviations and Units of Measurement

Neurodiagnostic Terminology

BAEP   Brainstem auditory evoked potential
BSAP   Brief small-amplitude polyphasic
CMAP   Compound motor action potential
EEG   Electroencephalography
EMG   Electromyography
EP   Evoked potential
MUP   Motor unit potential
NCV   Nerve-conduction velocity
SNAP   Sensory nerve action potential
SEP   Somatosensory evoked potential
VEP   Visual evoked potential

Muscles

The following abbreviations are routinely used by many electromyographers in annotating studies.

ADM   Abductor digiti minimi (or ADQ, abductor digiti
             quinti)
APB   Abductor pollicis brevis
EDB   Extensor digitorum brevis
EDC   Extensor digitorum communis
FDP   Flexor digitorum profundus (suffix is 1&2 or 3&4
             indicating median or ulnar innervated portions,
             respectively)
FDS   Flexor digitorum superficialis
1stDI   First dorsal interosseus
LG   Lateral gastrocnemius

MG	Medial gastrocnemius
RF	Rectus femoris
TA	Tibialis anterior
VM	Vastus medialis

Disorders

ALS	Amyotrophic lateral sclerosis
DMD	Duchenne muscular dystrophy
FSH	Facioscapulohumeral dystrophy
MG	Myasthenia gravis
MS	Multiple sclerosis
SMA	Spinal muscular atrophy

Units of Measurement

amp	Ampere
cm	Centimeter
dB	Decibels
Hz	Hertz
kHz	Kilohertz
kohm	Kilo-ohm (1,000 ohms)
mm	Millimeter
ms	Millisecond (0.001 second)
μs	Microsecond (0.000001 sec)
mV	Millivolt (0.001 volt)
μV	Microvolt (0.000001 volt)
sec	Second
V	Volts

Part

I

Basic Electronics

1

□ □ □
□ □ □
□ □ □

Theory of Electricity

Atomic Structure and Charge

Every atom has a nucleus composed of positively charged protons and uncharged neutrons. Negatively charged electrons orbit the nucleus. In most atoms, the number of electrons is equal to the number of protons in the nucleus, so that there is no net charge. If the number of electrons is less than the number of protons, then the atom has a net positive charge. If the number of electrons is greater than the number of protons, then the atom has a net negative charge. This is illustrated in Figure 1.1. The atom in *A* has full orbitals and no net charge. *B* has an empty orbital but still no charge. This atom could donate or accept an electron. *C* is the same atom as *A* but has lost an electron, giving it a charge of +1. *D* is the same atom as *B* but has filled its empty orbital with an electron, giving it a charge of –1. Within the universe, there is electrical neutrality; however, there are local concentrations of charge throughout biological and physical systems. These local concentrations are responsible for all electrical activity, from cellular membrane potentials to the power behind neurodiagnostic equipment.

Conductors, Semiconductors, and Nonconductors

Every atom can be induced to give up an electron, but the energy required differs greatly among atoms. Atoms that give up electrons easily can be conductors. Elements such as helium and silicon require so much energy to give up an electron that it almost never occurs in nature. They are nonconductors. Iron easily donates electrons and is stable at two different charge states, 2+ and 3+. Therefore, iron is an excellent conductor. Iron atoms have a loosely held electron and an empty electron orbital. With charge movement, iron accepts an electron and then releases it. Semiconductors are materials that can donate and accept electrons more easily than nonconductors but not as well as conductors. They are discussed in detail in chapter 4.

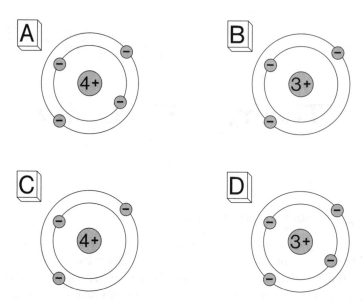

Figure 1.1   Diagram of atomic structure. The rings signify the outer orbitals. *A* has a full outer orbital and no net charge. *B* has one empty electron position but maintains electrical neutrality. This atom could easily accept an extra electron. Although it would give the atom a negative charge, the orbital would be filled. *C* has lost an electron and has 1+ charge. This is a stable state since there are no partially filled orbitals. *D* has accepted an electron and has a 1– charge. This is essentially the atom shown in *B* with the extra electron.

Figure 1.2 shows three views of a conductor. *A* is the atomic structure of the wire. The 3+ in the circle indicates the valence of the nucleus. The area encompassed by the arcs signifies the orbitals shared by adjacent atoms. Two electrons sharing an orbital is a very stable situation, even without electrical neutrality. The e symbols in the circles represent electrons filling some but not all orbital positions. The conductor is electrically neutral, which means that there is one electron for each nucleus valence. *B* is a somewhat less enlarged view of a conductor. This could be considered a magnified view of a wire, which is essentially a cylinder. A potential difference is applied across the conductor and electrons move in the direction indicated. *C* is a schematic of a conductor attached to a battery. (From this figure on, all electronic equipment is drawn in standard electronic schematic format.) Energy is imparted to the system to make electrons move from one atom to another. The energy required to make the electrons move may be obtained from a variety of sources, such as alternating current (AC) line voltage, a direct current (DC) battery, the electrochemical fluxes of a neuron, or a magnetic field. The driving force for electrons is a potential difference, which is measured in volts (V). The voltage causes electrons to flow through the wire from the negative terminal, through the wire, and into the positive terminal.

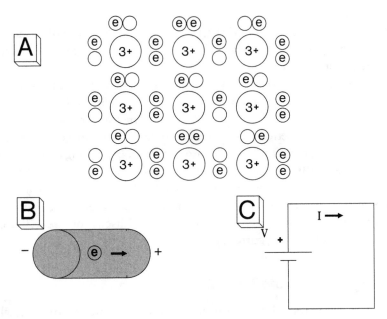

Figure 1.2 Diagram of a conductor. *A* is the atomic structure of a conductor with shared orbitals. The central circle with the number indicates the valence of the nucleus. The circles with the e symbols indicate electrons in the outer orbitals. Not all of the protons and electrons are shown. *B* is a somewhat less enlarged view. *C* is a schematic of a conductor connected to the terminals of a battery. The plus symbol indicates the positive terminal of the battery. Electrons flow from the negative terminal through the conductor to the positive terminal.

When no energy is applied to the conductor, electrons move randomly, with no net flow in any direction. When a potential difference is created through the wire by a power source, the electrons will have a net movement away from the negative side and toward the positive side.

The net movement of electrons through a conductor is current. Current *(I)* is the amount of charge *(Q)* moving through a conductor per unit time *(t)*. The unit of measurement of current is the ampere or amp. The unit of measurement of charge is the coulomb; 1 coulomb is equivalent to 6.24×10^{18} positive or negative charges. One amp of current is equivalent to the movement of 1 coulomb of charge per second through a conductor. Or:

$$I = Q/t$$

(Current = Charge/time)

We envision that electrons with high energy content flow out of the negative pole, through the wire, and into the positive pole. More accurately, the battery imparts energy to the electrons of the conductor in proximity to the negative pole. Thus, electrons are induced to leave their orbitals and flow toward the region of less negative charge, that is, the positive pole. There is a cascading action, with successive electrons in the conductor excited to travel toward the positive pole.

The flow of current was described earlier as the movement of negative charge. However, conventional terminology speaks of the flow of positive charge, which was designated before subatomic structure was understood. One can envision that if electrons are moving from left to right in a conductor, they are essentially skipping from atom to atom, temporarily filling empty orbitals. This is conceptually equivalent to having empty orbitals of atoms moving from right to left. Of course, this does not actually happen. The flow of positive charge is referred to as the flow of holes, which travel in the opposite direction to electron flow. For most of the rest of this discussion, we will use the convention of considering current as the flow of positive charge.

Electronic Equipment

Electronic equipment is composed of complex circuitry which can be broken down into functional modules. The basic modules are amplifiers, filters, stimulators, and displays. Each of these is discussed in subsequent chapters after a discussion of circuit theory in chapter 2. First, electrical characteristics of biological tissues are reviewed.

Electrical Properties of Biological Tissues

Ion Fluxes and Membrane Potentials

Nerve and muscle membranes conduct electricity in a fashion similar to that of wires. When recording from a patient, the tissues become an integral part of the circuit. Most of the charge movement in biological tissues can be attributed to passive properties of the membrane or to changes in ion conductance. The important positively charged ions are potassium (K^+), sodium (Na^+), and calcium (Ca^{+2}). The important negatively charged ions are chloride (Cl^-) and proteins ($Prot^-$). Positive ions are cations, while negative ions are anions.

Neuronal membrane has a resting potential of approximately -75 mV, due to differential permeability to ions. The sodium-potassium pump forces K^+ into the cell and Na^+ out of the cell. The pump itself is not electrogenic, that is, it does not cause a potential difference. The permeability to K^+ is greater than to any other ion. Therefore, K^+ diffuses out of the cell and down its chemical gradient. Anionic proteins cannot accompany the K^+ through the membrane, so the interior of the cell becomes negative compared to the exterior. The buildup of charge opposes the further efflux of K^+. When the charge is about −75 mV, the efflux of K$^+$ stops. This change is the equilibrium potential: the electrical gradient sufficient to prevent K$^+$ from flowing down its chemical gradient. The combination of electrical and chemical influences on an ion is its electrochemical gradient.

This description is for the equilibrium potential for K$^+$ (E_{K_+}), but the same principle can be applied to every ion. Permeability of the membrane to each ion is termed conductance (G). The contribution of each ion to the membrane potential is determined by its conductance. Since G_{K_+} is so much larger than G_{Na_+}, G_{Ca+2}, and so on, the resting membrane potential approximates E_{K_+}.

The Nernst equation describes the equilibrium potentials of ions as a function of their concentrations.

$$E_{Na} = -58 \log \frac{[Na]_i}{[Na]_o} \qquad \text{for sodium}$$

$$E_K = -58 \log \frac{[K]_i}{[K]_o} \qquad \text{for potassium}$$

$$E_{Cl} = -58 \log \frac{[Cl]_i}{[Cl]_o} \qquad \text{for chloride}$$

where E_{Na}, E_K, and E_{Cl} are the equilibrium potentials for sodium, potassium, and chloride, respectively, and the letters in brackets signify the concentrations of the respective ions. The i and o following the bracket indicate that the concentration is inside or outside of the cell.

The membrane potential depends on which ions have the greatest conductance. Since potassium has the greatest conductance at rest, then the resting membrane potential is closest to E_K, or −75 mV.

When an excitatory neurotransmitter activates the postsynaptic receptors, the conductance to sodium is increased. Therefore, the membrane potential approaches E_{Na}, approximately +45 mV.

Therefore, the membrane potential can be described as a function of the equilibrium potentials of individual ions weighted by the conductance to each ion. This relationship is described in the Goldman constant field equation:

$$V = -58 \log \frac{G_K[K]_i + G_{Na}[Na]_i + G_{Cl}[Cl]_i}{G_K[K]_o + G_{Na}[Na]_o + G_{Cl}[Cl]_o}$$

where G_K, G_{Na}, and G_{Cl} are the conductances to the individual ions, and the letters in brackets are the concentrations of the respective ions inside and outside of the cell. At rest, the conductance to potassium is so much greater than to any of the other ions that the equation is essentially the Nernst equation for potassium. During an action potential, the conductance to sodium is so great that the contributions of potassium and chloride to the equation are minimized.

Action Potentials

Action potentials develop in nerve and muscle fiber in response to depolarization. Neurotransmitters bind to the postsynaptic membrane receptors. These receptors open channels for the influx of sodium, thereby depolarizing the cell. An action potential only develops if the depolarization reaches threshold, which is determined by the voltage-dependent property of sodium channels. Depolarization causes the opening of additional sodium channels. With faster and greater depolarization, more and more channels open. Of course, each open channel further increases the conductance to sodium, producing further depolarization. There comes a point where the depolarization is sufficient to be regenerative. That is, a vicious cycle is established whereby depolarization produces more depolarization, and so on. This is threshold. The sodium conductance is so great that the membrane potential overshoots zero, becoming positive.

The sodium channels are not only voltage dependent, but also time dependent. *Time dependent* means that the channels can stay open only for a specified period of time. After that time they close, even though the cell is depolarized. With closure of the sodium channels, conductance to sodium declines, and the membrane potential once again approaches the equilibrium po-

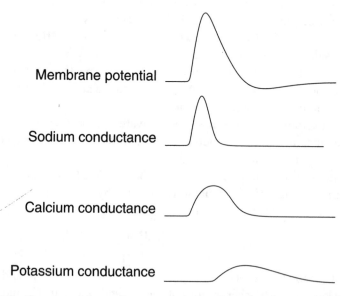

Figure 1.3   Sequence of membrane potential and ion conductances changes during an action potential. The initial phase of sodium conductance causes the depolarization. Calcium conductance increases, but at a slower rate than the sodium conductance. Potassium conductance subsequently increases, resulting in repolarization. Since the potassium conductance outlasts the drop in sodium conductance, there is some hyperpolarization of the membrane following the action potential.

tential of potassium. Figure 1.3 shows changes in membrane potential and ion conductances with an action potential. The second trace shows the changes in sodium conductance discussed in the previous section. The third trace is calcium conductance, which also is increased but is slower than the increase in sodium conductance. The last trace is potassium conductance. Since the chemical gradient for potassium favors efflux, the late increase in potassium conductance causes repolarization of the cell and even some hyperpolarization, as the membrane potential approaches the equilibrium potential for potassium.

Action potentials travel down an axon by serially depolarizing adjacent nodes. An action potential at one node produces depolarization of the next node. Under normal circumstances, this depolarization is always sufficient to produce an action potential at that point.

Generation of Electrical Activity by Nerve and Muscle

The generators of electroencephalographic (EEG) and electro–myographic (EMG) activity are discussed in detail in chapters 9 and 19. In general, the potentials recorded in clinical neurophysiologic studies have as origins (1) action potentials in nerve fiber bundles, whether they be peripheral nerves or central nerve tracts, and (2) extracellular potentials generated by movement of ions into and out of cells during depolarization and repolarization.

Field Potentials and Volume Conduction

The influx of sodium during an action potential is effectively an inward current. An intracellular electrode would see this as a positive potential, because the interior is becoming more positive than it was at rest. An extracellular electrode would see this as a negative potential because of the shift of positive charge from the extracellular space into the cell. The extracellular potential can be recorded at a considerable distance from the cell, which is known as a *field potential*. The movement of charge from excitable tissue through surrounding tissues is called *volume conduction*.

Field potentials are often described as near-field and far-field. Near-field potentials are recorded by electrodes close to the membrane, while far-field potentials are recorded at a distance. To illustrate, consider a peripheral nerve conducting a volley of action potentials. Refer to Figures 1.4, 1.5, and 1.6. The near-field potential can be recorded by a unipolar or bipolar recording arrangement. For a unipolar recording, the active electrode (G_1, for Grid 1, from tube terminology) is directly overlying the nerve and the reference (G_2) is on the same limb but not overlying the nerve (Figure 1.4). As the wave of depolarization passes under G_1, the inward current causes a prominent negative wave. As the wave passes, the potential returns to baseline.

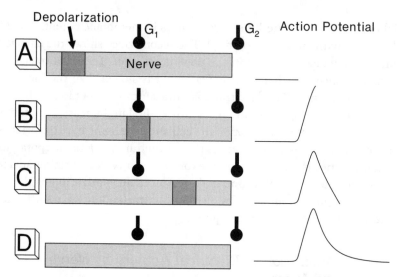

Figure 1.4 Unipolar near-field potential. This diagram should be compared with the two that follow. For each figure, the cascading figures show the effect of propagation of an action potential on the recording. The wave of depolarization travels from left to right. G_1 is the active electrode. G_2 is the reference and is not overlying the excitable membrane.

(A) Wave of depolarization has not yet reached the membrane under the electrode. *(B)* Maximal negativity occurs when the wave of depolarization is directly under the recording electrode. *(C)* The potential decays as it passes away from the active recording electrode. *(D)* The depolarization is long gone and the potential is back to baseline.

A bipolar recording is similar to a unipolar recording except that G_2 is over a distal segment of the nerve (Figure 1.5). The initial negative component is as previously described. However, as the depolarization passes under G_2, a positive phase occurs because the amplifier is measuring the difference in potential between G_1 and G_2. Depolarization at G_1 makes G_1 negative relative to G_2. Depolarization at G_2 makes G_2 negative relative to G_1, but this means that G_1 is positive relative to G_2. Therefore, the recording is biphasic.

The far-field potential is recorded with G_1 at a distance from the current generator, and G_2 at a greater distance, typically in a different tissue compartment (Figure 1.6). The far-field potential is a stationary wave that is due to the moving front of depolarization in the axons. Since the far-field potential is recorded at a distance, it is not governed by exact electrode position. If the nerve volley comes close to the active or reference electrode, a component of near-field potential may be seen.

Most of the potentials recorded in clinical neurophysiology are far-field potentials. The notable exception is the compound action potentials of nerve-conduction studies, which are largely near-field potentials.

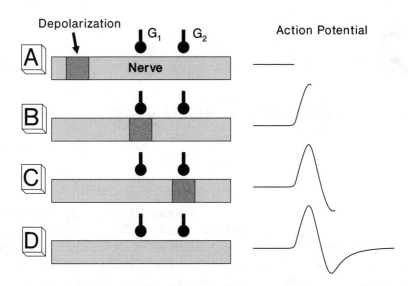

Figure 1.5 Bipolar near-field potential. Compare with Figures 1.4 and 1.6. The recording setup is similar to that of Figure 1.3 except that G_2 is located over a distal nerve segment. *(A)* The wave of depolarization has not yet reached the electrodes. *(B)* Maximal negativity occurs as the wave of depolarization passes under G_1. *(C)* Maximal positivity ensues as the wave of depolarization passes under G_2. *(D)* The depolarization is passed and the potential returns to baseline.

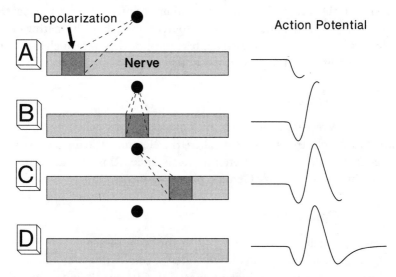

Figure 1.6 Far-field potential. Compare with Figures 1.4 and 1.5. G_1 is distant from the nerve. G_2 is not shown, and is located distant from G_1. *(A)* The advancing front of depolarization produces a positive far-field potential. *(B)* As the depolarization travels beneath the electrode, a negative potential is seen. *(C)* The receding phase of repolarization produces a following positive phase. *(D)* The potential has passed and the potential has returned to baseline.

2

□ □ □
□ □ □
□ □ □

Circuit Theory

A circuit is a closed loop or series of loops composed of circuit elements. Current requires a closed loop in order to flow; it will not flow into the blind end of a conductor. Circuit elements include power supplies, resistors, capacitors, inductors, and transistors. This chapter discusses circuit elements first and then presents the laws governing the function of electric circuits.

Circuit Elements

Power Supply

The power supply provides the energy to drive electrons (or holes) around the circuit. It produces a potential difference that the electrons flow down. Power can come from many sources, including alternating current (AC) line voltage, direct current (DC) batteries, or the voltage change across neuronal membranes. The potential difference is measured in volts (V).

Resistors

A resistor opposes the flow of electrons by converting the energy imparted to the electrons into heat. Thus, the electrons leaving a resistor have lost a considerable amount of energy. Resistance (R) is measured in ohms, after the nineteenth-century German physicist, Georg Ohm.

Capacitors

Capacitors store energy in the form of separation of charge. Briefly, a capacitor is made up of two plates of conducting material separated by a thin layer of a nonconducting material. Current flowing through the circuit results in the buildup of excess electrons on one plate and excess holes on the other plate. The dynamics of the charging and discharging of these plates is responsible for the frequency dependence of many electronic circuits. Therefore, the capacitor is a fundamental component of filters. A complete discussion of the theory of capacitors appears later in this chapter.

Inductors

Inductors store energy in the form of a magnetic field. Briefly, an inductor is a length of conducting wire that is wound into a very tight coil. The passage of current through the coil creates a strong magnetic field. This magnetic field can, in turn, influence the flow of current. The result is a complex relationship between the applied voltage and subsequent current. Inductors are included in most electronic equipment. The process of induction is especially important in the generation of noise. Inductors are discussed in more detail later in this chapter.

Semiconductors

Semiconductors are key elements of modern amplifiers and filters and are discussed in chapter 4. They conduct electricity better than nonconductors, but not as well as conventional conductors.

Laws Governing Circuit Theory

Ohm's Law

Ohm's law describes the relationship between current *(I)*, resistance *(R)*, and voltage *(V)* in a circuit or a circuit element:

$$V = I \times R$$

Ohm's law: The applied voltage is equal to the induced current times the resistance of the circuit.

This formula is mainly used to describe resistive circuits. Figure 2.1 shows a simple circuit that illustrates Ohm's law. The schematic at the top shows a resistor in series with a battery. The voltage of the battery *(V)* is equal to the induced current *(I)* times the resistance of the resistor *(R)*. The same general principle is operative with capacitors, although the resistance of capacitors is dependent on the frequency of the applied voltage below. The formula $V = I \times R$ may not seem intuitively obvious, but the relationship becomes clearer when permutations of the formula are considered (see Figure 2.1):

1. When resistance is fixed, the applied voltage and resulting current have a direct relationship. Therefore, an increase in applied voltage produces a proportionately greater current flow.
2. When voltage is constant, resistance and current have an inverse relationship. Therefore, an increase in resistance produces a reduction in current.

Ohm's law is the basis by which other circuit laws are derived.

Kirchoff's Current Law

A node is a junction point of two or more conductors. Figure 2.2A shows one junction point (node) in a circuit. The loops of the circuit are all complete, but the remainder of the elements making up the circuit are not shown. I_1, I_2, and I_3 are the currents flowing through the three wires into and out of the node.

The node has no capacity to store or produce energy and has no ability to alter energy imparted to it. Therefore, the sum of all the current flowing into a node equals the current flowing out. Expressed mathematically:

$$I_1 = I_2 + I_3$$

or, rearranging,

$$I_1 - I_2 - I_3 = 0.$$

Since the currents flowing out of the node are actually negative currents (meaning opposite in direction, not opposite in charge), then

$$I_1 + I_2 + I_3 = 0.$$

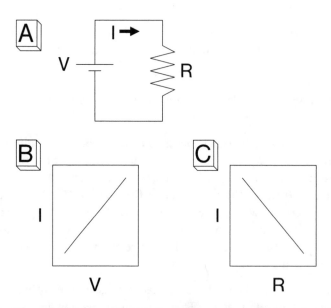

Figure 2.1   Ohm's law. *A* is a simple circuit diagram of a resistor in series with a battery. By Ohm's law, the voltage of the battery (V) is equal to the current (I) times the resistance of the resistor (R) ($V = I \times R$). While Ohm's law applies to this simple circuit, it is defined to apply to the voltage dissipated by individual resistors within more complex circuits. *B* is a graph showing the relationship between voltage and current. *C* is a graph showing the relationship between resistance and current.

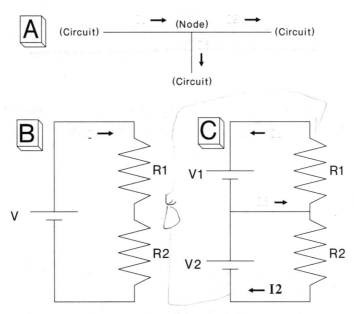

Figure 2.2 Kirchoff's laws. *(A)* Kirchoff's current law. This is a schematic of the junction point of three conductors. I_1, I_2, and I_3 are the currents in each conductor. The current flowing into the node must equal the current flowing out. *(B)* Kirchoff's voltage law. A battery is in series with two resistors, R_1 and R_2. The voltage applied must be equal to the sum of the voltage drops across the two resistors. *(C)* Kirchoff's voltage law applies to each of the three potential loops in this schematic: (1) the upper loop with battery V_1 and resistor R_1, (2) the lower loop with battery V_2 and resistor R_2, and (3) the large loop encompassing both batteries and both resistors.

There may be any number of conductors coming into a node. The sum of all of the currents coming into and out of the node must be zero, so

$$\Sigma I = 0.$$

Kirchoff's current law: For any node, the sum of the currents flowing into and out of the node is zero.

Kirchoff's Voltage Law

For any loop of a circuit, the energy imparted to the loop must equal the energy dissipated. This makes sense, since the circuit elements uses all available power coming from the power source.

Figure 2.2B shows a battery forming a circuit loop with two resistors in series. The energy is imparted by the battery (V), and the voltage is dissipated by resistors R_1 and R_2. Current (I) flows from the battery through the two resistors. Since there is only one path, the current is equal through all portions of the loop. If the current is multiplied by the resistance of one of the resistors (R_1), the product is called the *voltage drop* across the resistor (V_1). This is an adaptation of Ohm's law $(V = I \times R)$, where the voltage drop across a resistor is equal to the resistance of the resistor (in ohms) multiplied by the current flowing through the resistor (in amps).

Kirchoff's voltage law can be reworded: For any circuit loop, the sum of the voltage sources is equal to the sum of the voltage drops. Expressed mathematically:

$$V_t + V_1 + V_2 = 0$$

or

$$V_t = (V_1)(V_2)$$

$$\Sigma V = 0$$

for any loop.

> *Kirchoff's voltage law:* For any circuit loop, the sum of the voltage sources is equal to the sum of the voltage drops.

Kirchoff's voltage law applies to any loop, even though it may be part of a larger circuit. In Figure 2.2C, Kirchoff's voltage law applies to both the top and bottom loops. In fact, it also applies to the large loop that encompasses both batteries and both resistors.

Theory of Resistors

Resistors impede the flow of electrons through a circuit. Energy is dissipated because resistors convert the energy imparted to the electrons by the power supply into heat. Since the electrons have less associated energy, they flow less forcefully down their electrical gradient toward ground. Therefore, resistors decrease the effective voltage of the electrons, that is, a voltage drop occurs.

If the two terminals of a battery are connected by a wire (Figure 2.3A), a massive flow of current between the terminals would quickly destroy the battery. However, if a resistor is placed in the wire (Figure 2.3B), some of the energy imparted to the electrons would be converted to heat and fewer electrons would flow to the positive terminal. The current would be reduced.

Series Resistance

If current runs through two or more resistors connected serially, energy will be dissipated by both resistors. In Figure 2.3C, V is the total voltage delivered to the battery, I is the current through the entire circuit, R_1 and R_2 are the resistances of the two resistors, and V_1 and V_2 the voltage drops across the

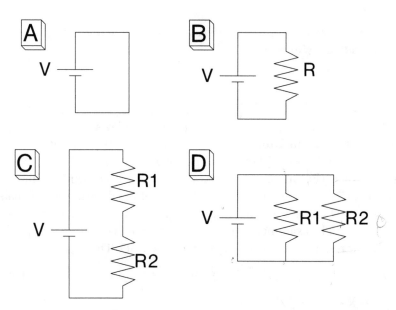

Figure 2.3 Theory of resistors. *(A)* The terminals of a battery are connected by a wire, resulting in a massive but brief flow of current. Current stops as the battery is discharged. *(B)* The leads of a resistor are connected to the terminals of the battery. Current flows from the positive terminal through the resistor and into the negative terminal. Energy is dissipated at the resistor as heat. *(C)* Two resistors are connected in series. The total resistance of the circuit in *C* can be represented as an equivalent resistance (Req). This would look like diagram *B* with R being Req. *(D)* Two resistors are connected in parallel. The total resistance can be represented as an equivalent resistance as for *C*.

two resistors. Figure 2.3D shows the same circuit with the serial resistors represented as a single equivalent resistance. The purpose of this exercise is to determine the equivalent resistance of the two resistors connected in series.

From Ohm's law:

$$V_1 = I \times R_1 \quad \text{and} \quad V_2 = I \times R_2$$

since

$$V = V_1 + V_2 \qquad \text{(Kirchoff's voltage law)}$$

and the equivalent resistance of the system $Req = V/I$, then

$$Req = \frac{(I \times R_1) + (I \times R_2)}{I} = R_1 + R_2$$

Thus, for series resistances,

$$Req = \Sigma R.$$

For resistors in series, the total resistance is equal to the sum of the individual resistances.

Parallel Resistance

In a circuit with branch points, the laws for circuit loops still apply, and they apply for each loop. In Figure 2.3D, the total current (I) traveling from the (+) to (–) terminals of the battery splits into the two parallel resistor arms. The amount of current down each path depends on the relative resistances. From Kirchoff's voltage law, the voltage drop across R_1 equals that across R_2 and equals the imparted voltage (V), since there are three circuit loops that can be examined. The parallel resistances can be represented by an equivalent resistance termed *Req* as in Figure 2.3D. Thus,

$$V_1 = I_1 \times R_1 \text{ and } V_2 = I_2 \times R_2 \qquad \text{(Ohm's law) } \textbf{(2.1)}$$

rearranging

$$I_1 = V_1/R_1 \text{ and } I_2 = V_2/R_2, \qquad \textbf{(2.2)}$$

since

$$It = I_1 + I_2 \qquad \text{(Kirchoff's current law) } \textbf{(2.3)}$$

substituting equation (2.2) into equation (2.3)

$$V/Rt = V_1/R_1 + V_2/R_2 \qquad \textbf{(2.4)}$$

but we know that

$$V_1 = V \text{ and } V_2 = V \quad \text{(Kirchoff's voltage law) } \textbf{(2.5)}$$

substituting equation (2.5) into (2.4)

$$V/Rt = V/R_1 + V/R_2 \qquad \textbf{(2.6)}$$

V drops out from both sides of equation (2.6), so

$$1/Rt = 1/R_1 + 1/R_2 \qquad \textbf{(2.7)}$$

or

$$1/Rt = \Sigma \, 1/Ri \qquad \text{for parallel resistances. } \textbf{(2.8)}$$

For resistors in parallel, the total resistance is equal to the reciprocal of the sum of the reciprocals of the individual resistances.

One corollary of this formula is that total resistance is always less than any of the individual resistances. This makes sense because, for any resistor, if you provide an additional pathway electrons will find the path "easier." To illustrate, consider this analogy: if a small hole is placed in the bottom of a bucket, a small stream of water will flow out through the high resistance. If there are two small holes, the flow will be substantially faster, even though each hole has relatively high resistance.

Conductance is the reciprocal of resistance. For any resistor, if the resistance to flow of electrons is high, then it is less able to conduct electrons, hence, the conductance is less. If there are several resistors in parallel (or several holes in the bucket), then the total conductance (G) is equal to the sum of the individual conductances. Expressed mathematically:

$$Gt = G_1 + G_2 + G_3 + \ldots$$

where Gt is the total conductance, and G_1, G_2, and G_3 are the conductances of the individual resistors. Since conductance is the reciprocal of resistance:

$$1/Rt = 1/R_1 + 1/R_2 + 1/R_3 + \ldots$$

This is the same formula we derived above.

Theory of Capacitors

Capacitors store energy by separating electrons (–) from holes (+). They are composed of two thin plates of conducting material separated by a very thin layer of nonconducting material. Figure 2.4A shows an electrical diagram of a capacitor. Wires are attached to the two plates for connection with the rest of the circuit, which in this case consists only of a battery. Figure 2.4B is a closeup of the same capacitor showing electrons flowing onto one side of the plate from the negative terminal of the battery, while holes flow onto the other side from the positive terminal. Actually, on the positive side, electrons flow off the plate and into the positive terminal, leaving holes.

Considering this structure, it is evident that electrons cannot flow through the capacitor, since they cannot jump the thin gap between the plates. Because the plates are so close, electrons sent to one plate repel electrons on the other plate, making them travel out the other wire. Thus, electrons can flow onto one plate, which in turn causes electrons to flow off of the next, producing an apparent current flow through the capacitor, although the current is not being carried by the same electrons. This current is a capacitative current, since no electrons actually complete the journey through the capacitor. Capacitative current results in a buildup of voltage across the capacitor; subsequently, the negative charge on one plate counterbalances the potential difference of the power supply. When the voltage across the capacitor plates is equal to but opposite from the voltage of the power supply, the negative charge on one plate prevents any more electrons from leaving and the flow of electrons stops.

Figure 2.4C shows the capacitor once the potential difference is turned off (the complete circuit is not shown). The potential difference across the capacitor forces electrons off one side of the plates and holes off the other. Or, in other words, electrons flow off the plate that has an excess of electrons,

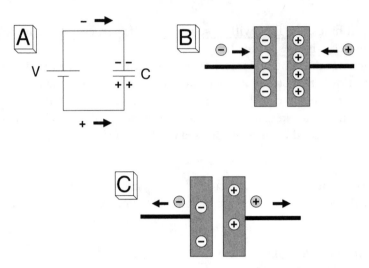

Figure 2.4   Theory of capacitors. *(A)* A capacitor is connected to the terminals of a battery. Charge flows from the battery onto the plates of the capacitor. Current flow stops when the charge on the capacitor is equal to and opposite the charge of the battery. *(B)* Close-up of the plates of the capacitor with the leads to the battery on the right and left sides. Circles with (+) symbols indicate movement of "holes," while circles with (–) symbols indicate movement of electrons. *(C)* When the potential difference is abolished, the holes and electrons stream off of the plates. This requires an intact circuit, not shown.

through the circuit, and onto the plate with a deficit of electrons (excess holes), thereby filling the holes and discharging the voltage across the capacitor. Thus, following cessation of applied voltage, there is reversal of flow of current due to energy imparted to electrons from the voltage built up across the capacitor.

The characteristics of a capacitor depend on its capacitance (C), measured in farads (after Michael Faraday, an eighteenth-century English chemist and physicist). This property reflects how much charge can be built up on a capacitor for a given voltage. If the capacity (capacitance) is low because the plates are small, then a relatively high voltage will be built up after very little current flow. In contrast, if the capacitance is large, then much more current must flow onto (and off) the plates in order to develop a comparable voltage. Expressed mathematically:

$$I = k(dV/dt)$$

where k is a proportionality constant that represents the capacitance of the capacitor. Thus,

$$I = C(dV/dt).$$

In other words, the capacitative current is proportional to the rate of change of voltage. This is an important concept. The implication of this relationship is that capacitative current is frequency dependent—a factor used in designing high- and low-frequency filters (filters will be discussed in the next section). Capacitance is also important in generation of noise in neurodiagnostic recordings, which are discussed in chapter 7.

Theory of Inductors

Inductors store energy in the form of a magnetic field created by the movement of charge, similar to the energy stored in a capacitor by the potential difference between separated positive and negative charges. When current flows through a wire, it produces a weak magnetic field that is oriented circumferentially to the wire (see Figure 2.5). An inductor consists of a coil of conducting wire with two leads incorporated into a circuit. When current flows through the wire, the coiling makes the magnetic fields orient in the same direction, along the axis of the coil. The influence of the magnetic field on the flow of electrons is to oppose a change in current. Current through an inductor cannot change instantaneously. If the voltage is increased, some of the additional energy will also increase the magnetic field. Therefore, current does not build up as much as would be expected without an inductor in the circuit. If current is decreased (by reducing the voltage), some of the energy in the magnetic field will be imparted to electrons in the conducting coil, thereby transiently maintaining current. This is because the greatest effect on the flow of electrons is not the presence of a magnetic field, but the change in a magnetic field. The process of induction, an important cause of noise in neurodiagnostic recordings, will be discussed in chapter 7.

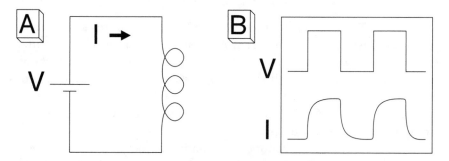

Figure 2.5 Theory of inductors. *A* is a diagrammatic representation of an inductor. A coil of wire is connected to the circuit by the two ends of the wire. A magnetic field is oriented along the axis indicated by the arrow. *B* is a graph of the effects of changing applied voltage on current through an inductor. An inductor resists changes in current.

3

□ □ □
□ □ □
□ □ □

Filters

All biological signals can be broken down into fundamental frequencies, with each frequency having its own intensity. Display of the intensities of all frequencies is called a power spectrum. In clinical neurophysiology, we are usually interested in signals of a particular frequency range or band width. The band width differs for individual studies. Other frequencies are less informative and may actually obscure important information. Therefore, unwanted frequencies are filtered out of the display. Figure 3.1 shows how a biological signal is composed of its fundamental frequencies; *A* shows how a high-frequency signal, such as spikes, can be added to a low-frequency signal, such as a sine wave, to produce a complex waveform; *B* shows power spectra for the corresponding signals. The complex signal is composed of both high- and low-frequency components.

Filters can be active or passive. Active filters use exogenous energy to alter the waveform, while passive filters do not. We will discuss passive filters first. Fundamental to the passive filter is the resistor-capacitor (RC) circuit.

RC Circuits and Passive Filters

The key to filter theory is the RC circuit, or resistor/capacitor circuit, as illustrated in Figure 3.2A. A resistor *(R)* and capacitor *(C)* are in series with a power source that is the signal voltage *(Vs)*. The effects of a sudden change in voltage (called *step voltage*) on current and voltage drops across the resistor and capacitor are illustrated in 3.2B. Immediately, current *(I)* begins to flow. As current flows, a voltage difference develops between the two terminals of the resistor (since $Vr = I \times R$). This current also results in a buildup of charge on the capacitor as capacitative current flows. The charge on the capacitor opposes the flow of further current, ultimately stopping flow when the voltage on the charged capacitor is equal and opposite to the applied signal voltage. When no current is flowing, there is no voltage across the resistor ($Vr = I \times R$ with $I =$ O).

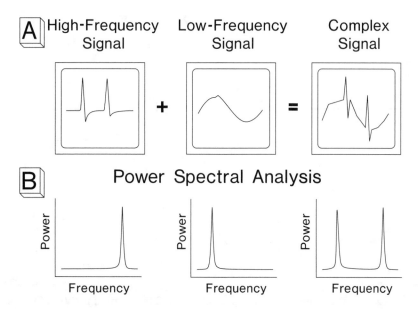

Figure 3.1 Frequency components of biologic signals. *(A)* Diagrammatic representation of oscilloscope traces of a complex signal. The left diagram shows a signal composed mainly of fast frequencies. The middle shows a signal composed of a slow wave. The right trace is the summation of the two. *(B)* Power spectral analysis of the signals shown in the simulated oscilloscope traces. Summed signal can be represented as a sum of the power spectral analysis. Or, a complex signal can be decomposed into fundamental frequencies.

When the voltage is suddenly decreased to baseline, the only source of current is the charged capacitor. Electrons flow off the lower plate toward the battery. Likewise, electrons from the battery flow through the conductor and through the resistor to occupy the holes on the upper plate. Current is flowing opposite to the direction it was flowing when the voltage was applied.

In summary, when there is a sudden change in voltage, the voltage is high across the resistor and low across the capacitor. As voltage increases on the capacitor, the voltage across the resistor decreases exponentially and eventually falls to zero as the current stops.

For the capacitor:

$$I = C \times dV/dt$$

where C is the capacitance and dV/dt is the change in voltage with time.

Since, in Figure 3.2A, the voltage across the capacitor *(Vc)* represents the cumulative flow of charge onto the plates, then *Vc* is inversely proportional to the capacitance and directly proportional to the total amount of charge that has gone onto the plate (that is, the integral of current with respect to time).

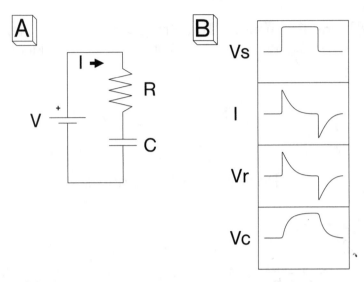

Figure 3.2　Resistor-capacitor (RC) circuit. *A* is a schematic diagram of the resistor and capacitor connected in series to a battery. The formula for Vr is Ohm's law. The formula for Vc is the formula for voltage across a capacitor. *B* shows the effects of a step voltage on current and voltage drops across the resistor and capacitor. The resistor has a voltage across it only when current is flowing. The capacitor develops a potential between the plates which is proportional to the total charge flowing onto the plates.

Or

$$Vc = (1/C) \times \int I \, dt.$$

For the resistor

$$Vr = I \times R \qquad\qquad \text{(Ohm's law)}$$

since

$$I = C \times dV/dt$$

then

$$Vr = R \times C \times dV/dt.$$

This means that (1) the voltage drop across the resistor *(Vr)* is greatest when the signal voltage *(Vs)* is changing, and (2) the voltage across the capacitor *(Vc)* is greatest when the signal voltage is not changing (at steady state). In other words, if we are looking at the voltage across the two elements of the circuit, the resistor responds to changes in voltage and cuts out low frequencies, whereas the capacitor responds to steady-state voltages and cuts out high frequencies.

　　This is the basis for high- and low-frequency filters. The signal is applied across an RC circuit with an amplifier looking at the voltage across either the resistor or the capacitor. If the amplifier is looking at the voltage across the capacitor, the device is a high-frequency filter (HFF), whereas if the amplifier is looking at the voltage across the resistor the device is a low-frequency filter (LFF). Electrical devices use HFFs and LFFs in tandem to eliminate the high and low ends of the frequency spectrum.

The voltage of a battery that is being turned on and off is essentially a square-wave pulse that has both high- and low-frequency components: a slow-frequency step component and a fast-frequency phasic component, representing the rise and fall of the step (as the switch is turned on and off). In reality, biological signals are complex and are made up of a mixture of fast and slow frequencies.

The exponential rate at which current and voltage rise and fall in an RC circuit is described by the time constant (TC). The time constant, measured in seconds, is the time required for a step voltage to charge the capacitor to within 37% of the signal voltage. The 37% figure is derived from the reciprocal of the natural logarithm, e, which is about 2.7 ($1/e = 0.37$, or 37%). The time constant is dependent on the resistance and capacitance of the RC circuit. The larger the capacitance, the longer current will have to flow in order to charge the capacitor. The larger the resistance, the less current will flow, again requiring a longer time to charge the capacitor. In other words, the time constant is directly proportional to both the capacitance *(C)* and resistance *(R)*. Thus

$$TC = k \times R \times C$$

where *TC* is the time constant and *k* is a proportionality constant.

Since this is an exponential function and we defined TC as the time to $1/e$ of maximum, then the proportionality constant drops out, leaving

$$TC = R \times C.$$

Using this relationship, filters of the desired time constants are selected, allowing passage of the appropriate frequency band to the amplifier while rejecting the others. Separate time constants are selected for both the high- and low-frequency filters, so that the appropriate band width is selected.

High-frequency filters look at Vc, and
Low-frequency filters look at Vr.

Figure 3.3A illustrates the effect of varying the time constant on the voltage profiles developed across a resistor *(Vr)* and capacitor *(Vc)*. The limitation of the voltage profiles imposed by the selected filters is the frequency response curve.

Figure 3.3B shows the effect of changing the time constant on the power spectrum allowed by the filters. Effects on both high- and low-frequency filters

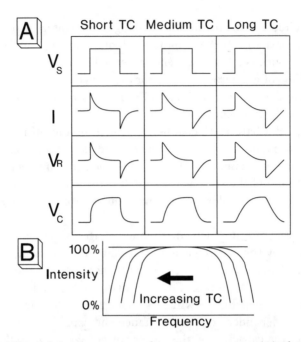

Figure 3.3   Effect of time constant on frequency response. *(A)* Changes in response to a step voltage with different time constants. *(B)* Frequency response curves with differing time constants. While the term *time constant* is usually used to indicate the response of the low-frequency filter, change in time constant governs response of the high-frequency filter.

are shown. The half-amplitude frequency is the frequency for either high- or low-frequency filters in which the ratio of output to input voltage has fallen by one-half (6 decibels [dB]). The term *turnover frequency* refers to the frequency at which the decrease in frequency response has fallen to approximately 70% (3 dB) from the maximum. Below the turnover frequency, the rate of decrease is accelerated. The speed of this decline is termed the *roll-off* and is expressed as dB/octave. For example, the roll-off may be 6 dB/octave, that is, the response is cut in half (6 dB) for each octave change in frequency. For both high- and low-frequency filters this frequency can be calculated from the resistance and capacitance of the circuit by the following formula:

$$70\% \text{ frequency} = \frac{1}{2\pi RC}$$

An example of the use of this formula is the determination of turnover frequency of machines in which the low-frequency filter specification is given as time constant rather than frequency. Most electroencephalography (EEG) machines represent the low-frequency filter settings by the time constant, since this is easy to measure on the calibration pulses. In contrast, Grass machines use the 80% frequency to specify the setting of the low-frequency filter (the frequency at the low end of the frequency response curve at which the output has fallen to 80% of maximum). Most EEG machines represent the high-frequency filter by the 3dB (70%) frequency. Grass instruments use the 80% frequency (the frequency at the upper end of the frequency response curve at which the signal has fallen to 80% of control).

Active Filters

Active filters require energy to modify the input waveform. They are composed of an amplifier, plus other circuit elements. Feedback loops reduce the amplification of signals that are above or below a specified frequency. A power supply, such as a battery or transformer, drives the amplifier. The principles of frequency-dependent response is the same as that described for passive filters, but the circuitry is much more complex.

Most equipment used in clinical neurophysiology uses active filters. It is not important to understand circuit schematics of active filters. Rather, it is more important to grasp the concepts of frequency response and the fundamentals of filter theory.

Digital Filters

Analog-to-digital (A/D) conversion is discussed in chapter 4; however, digital filtering will be considered briefly here. The computer converts the analog signal into digital format after some preamplification and filtering. Digital filters do not compensate for the distortions in the signal made by previous analog filters. However, digital filters allow for further modification of the signal.

Digital filters are essentially calculations performed on the digitized data. A common method of digitally filtering is to perform a Fourier transformation of a segment of data, reduce the value of selected frequencies, and then compute the inverse Fourier transformation. Other methods use interrelationships between data points in complex calculations that will not be discussed here.

The effects of digital filtering are difficult to represent graphically, and even more difficult to understand conceptually. Digital filtering does not result in a smooth frequency-response curve, as with analog filters.

One specific type of digital filter does not produce the phase distortions characteristic of analog filters; however, a frequently employed digital filter does. The commonly held belief that all digital filters prevent phase distortions is incorrect.

60-Hertz (Notch) Filters

EEG machines have a 60-Hz filter, sometimes referred to as a _notch filter_. This serves to subtract out activity in the 60-Hz range (the frequency of line power), thus removing artifact from line voltage affecting the recording electrodes. However, the 60-Hz filter does cut some frequency response slightly above and below 60 Hz.

Using the 60-Hz filter during recording of EEG activity can distort the recording of muscle activity, making it resemble beta activity. Therefore, this filter should not be used to compensate for 60-Hz noise caused by high-electrode impedances.

4

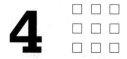

✓ Amplifiers

Amplifiers are integral to all equipment used in clinical electrophysiology. Transistors are the critical component of modern amplifiers. They replaced vacuum tubes, which had a limited life span and were much more expensive to make. Most amplification is performed by integrated circuits or "chips," wafers that contain many components in complex circuits.

Transistors

Transistors are a class of semiconductors. Understanding semiconductors is essential to understanding transistors and amplifiers.

Semiconductor Theory

Semiconductors are poorer conductors than some materials but are better than others, that is, they "semi-conduct." The solid materials that make up semiconductors do not conduct as well as most metals, having less loosely held electrons, or less "holes." Silicon and germanium, which normally have very low conductance, are doped with impurities in order to increase the numbers of holes and electrons available for movement in an electric field. The doping process controls the degree of conductance.

Doping the tetravalent base material (silicon or germanium, Figure 4.1A) with a pentavalent element (such as arsenic) results in one electron being held less tightly than the others, so that it is available for conduction of charge (Figure 4.1B). Since the loosely held charge is negative, this is referred to as an *N-doped material*. If, on the other hand, the material is doped with a trivalent element (such as gallium), the absence of sufficient electrons to fill all of the orbitals will leave a hole or place of deficiency of an electron, even though there is actually electrical neutrality (Figure 4.1C). This is *P-doped material*. Thus, N-doped materials have electrons available for movement, whereas P-doped materials have areas that have a potential space for electrons.

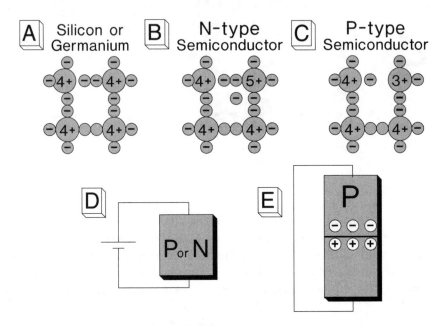

Figure 4.1 Semiconductors. *(A)* Parent structure of semiconductors. This matrix of tetravalent atoms is essentially a nonconductor. *(B)* N-doped semiconductor. The pentavalent atom has an "extra" electron that is available to conduct current. *(C)* P-type semiconductor. The trivalent atom causes a hole in the electron orbitals which can accept electrons moving in transit as current. *(D)* Semiconductor connected to a battery. Current will flow regardless of whether the semiconductor is N-type or P-type. *(E)* An N-P junction. Some electrons from the N-doped side will cross into the P-doped side and fill the empty orbitals. This migration progresses until the charge built up across the junction is sufficient to inhibit further movement of electrons.

Current can flow either way through N- or P-type semiconductor material. If a battery is connected to two ends of the material, electrons will flow in and a corresponding number of electrons will flow out (Figure 4.1D).

The useful properties of semiconductors appear when two or more dissimilar semiconductors are adjacent (Figure 4.1E). This figure shows adjacent N and P semiconductor materials. When these materials are placed together, electrons diffuse from the N region to the P region, filling some of the empty orbitals of the P region; this occurs until the relative attraction of the empty orbitals of the P material for electrons is counterbalanced by a charge differential built up across the junction. This is very similar to the physiological basis for the resting membrane potential in neural tissue. In NP junctions as well as neural membranes, an electrical field is built up at the junction that establishes an equilibrium with the driving force for flow of electrons.

If voltage is applied so that positive current flows into the P region and

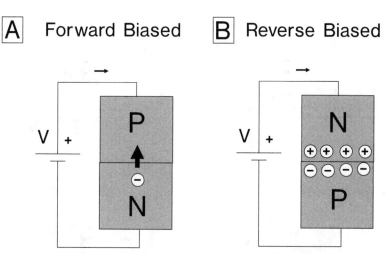

| A | Forward Biased | B | Reverse Biased |

Figure 4.2 Diode function. *(A)* Forward-biased junction. Current can flow since the applied potential dissipates the junction potential, allowing more electrons to cross the junction. Electrons flow from N to P. The arrow indicates the flow of positive current. *(B)* Reverse-biased junction. The applied potential only accentuates the junction potential, preventing flow of current. In the region of the junction, the N-doped material is depleted of electrons, while the P-doped material has the orbitals filled.

negative current into the N region, then the electrical field built up at the junction of the semiconductors is reduced and current can flow (Figure 4.2A). If, on the other hand, positive voltage is applied at the N region, the diffusion potential is augmented and the flow of current is blocked (Figure 4.2B), because the electrons from the N material have crossed to the other side of the junction to fill the empty orbitals of the P material and are unavailable for conduction of current. Similarly, the holes of the P material near the junction are filled. Thus, this junction allows for conduction only in one direction; the junction is a functioning diode. If the voltage applied across the semiconductor junction results in flow of current, it is *forward biased*; if the voltage is applied in the opposite direction, so that no current flows, it is *reverse biased.*

Transistors

The term *transistor* is derived from the words *transfer* and *resistor*, since the transistor controls the transference of energy across a resistance. Transistors work like vacuum tubes in older electrophysiological equipment do. In both tubes and transistors, a small gating current controls the flow of much greater current along another pathway. This is analogous to an automobile, where the relatively small amount of force applied to the gas pedal by the driver's foot proportionately controls the much greater force of the engine.

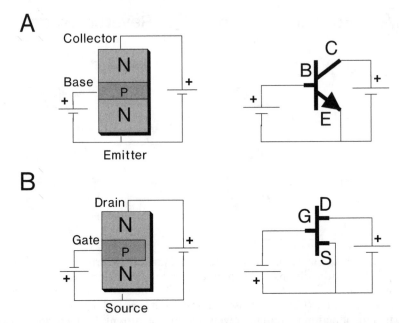

Figure 4.3 Transistor construction. For both sections of this figure, a diagram illustrating composition is on the left, and a schematic is on the right. *(A)* Field-effect transistor. Potential applied across the gate and source controls current flow between the drain and source. An applied potential blocks conduction through the thin N segment. No free electrons are available for conduction. *(B)* Junction bipolar transistor. Potential applied across the base and emitter controls current flow from the collector to emitter. The upper junction is reverse biased and will not conduct, but with applied potential, the "excess" electrons are removed, allowing current to flow.

There are several types of transistors, but they essentially operate on the same principle. Schematic diagrams of a field-effect transistor (FET) and a junction bipolar transistor are shown in Figure 4.3. Both have three connections to the transistor. Conductance between two of the terminals (drain and source, or emitter and collector) is influenced by the voltage bias delivered across the third (the gate or base). In transistors, a small controlling voltage can gate the flow of electrons through a circuit with larger voltage by changing the resistance of the transistor. Therefore, amplification is one of the most common uses for transistors.

The junction bipolar transistors are of two types, *NPN* and *PNP*. The letters refer to the configuration of the three-layer sandwich that makes up the transistor, where N stands for negative and P stands for positive, as detailed in the preceding section on semiconductors. Thus, the NPN has positively doped material in the middle layer, whereas PNP has negatively doped material in the middle layer. For either type of junction bipolar transistor, the controlling terminal is the base, and the controlled current flows between the emitter and collector.

For an NPN bipolar junction transistor (Figure 4.3A), the base-emitter P–lower N junction is forward biased, so that current can flow. In contrast, the pathway through the transistor from emitter to collector includes the reverse-biased upper N-P junction, as well as the forward-biased P–lower N junction. Therefore, little current will flow in the collector-emitter circuit. However, when voltage is applied across the base and emitter and the electrical barrier between P and lower N is reduced, the barrier between P and upper N is reduced as well. This is because the equilibrium potential at upper N-P, which normally prevents current flow, is reduced by electrons on the P side of the junction that are being sucked off into the base, leaving available holes. As a result, conduction between the collector and emitter is facilitated. The way the transistor is designed, the base P material is very thin, so only a very small base-emitter voltage must be applied to facilitate large conductances between collector and emitter. Thus, controlling voltage across base and emitter governs conductance of a much greater voltage applied across the collector and emitter. This is the basis of amplification using the junction bipolar transistor.

Field-effect transistors function similarly to bipolar junction transistors, but the movement of charge is somewhat different. FETs transform a small increase in controlling voltage to a large decrease in controlled current (Figure 4.3B). In this case, the gate-source junction (controlling circuit) is reverse biased, so that virtually no current flows through the junction when voltage is applied. In contrast to the junction bipolar transistor, the FET has a drain and source of contiguous N-type materials that allow unobstructed current flow. However, as voltage is applied across the gate-source circuit, the region of depletion of electrons and holes (at the junction of the N and P regions) is enhanced. This effect is most pronounced at the thin connecting segment between the drain and source. Carriers of charge are removed from this segment. Within a certain range this effect is proportional. Therefore, whereas this action is similar to that of the junction bipolar transistor, the effect is actually opposite in sign, that is, increasing gate-source voltage decreases drain-source conductance.

Amplifiers

Amplifiers are quite complex compared to RC circuits and transistors. However, their function is conceptually easy to understand; they magnify the signal so that it can be displayed. Figure 4.4A shows a schematic diagram of the pathway of electrical information from the patient to display. Shortly after the biological signal enters the electrophysiological device, and before any signal processing takes place, a preamplifier boosts the signal.

There are two reasons for preamplification: (1) so that the filters have sufficient signal voltage to deal with; and (2) so that the level of signal voltage is much higher than that of system noise.

The filters are positioned after the preamplifier to exclude unwanted information before the signal is sent to the driver amplifier. The function of the driver amplifier is to increase the signal intensity sufficiently to drive a chart pen or oscilloscope beam. Both amplifiers require an exogenous power source whose output is controlled by the signal voltage.

Figure 4.4B shows a transistor circuit with a signal voltage that varies between 0 and 1 V. The signal voltage controls conductance through the right side of the circuit, so that the output impedance sees proportionately between 0 and 10 V of a 20 V output power supply (Figure 4.4C). The gain of this simple amplifier is 10×. Depending on the size of the output power supply, the potential gain could potentially be much larger. However, semiconductors break down at high differential voltages so the amplification of each amplifier stage

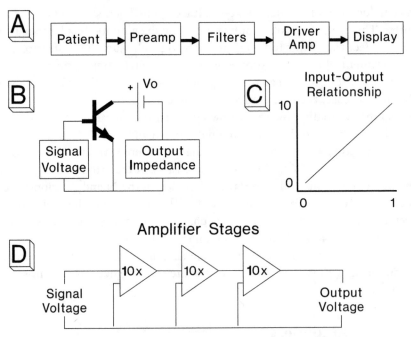

Figure 4.4 Amplifiers. *(A)* Pathway of signal movement from patient ultimately to the display of the apparatus. *(B)* Schematic of a single-stage amplifier. Vo is the output power supply of the amplifier. The signal voltage controls the impedance to flow through the resistor. This controls current through the right side of the circuit. The voltage drop across the output impedance is greater than the input voltage. *(C)* Input-output relationship of the amplifier shown in *B*. *(D)* Three-stage amplifier. Each stage represents approximately 10× gain, for a net gain of 103 or 1000×.

is fixed at 9×. For example, in order to get a gain of 1000×, at least three stages must be used. Thus, the amplifier stages are placed in series, as in Figure 4.4D.

Ideally, each amplifier stage should draw minimal current from the preceding stage. Otherwise, amplification is decreased and the signal may be distorted. The distortion is due to frequency-dependent effects of the amplifier-to-amplifier connection, by virtue of capacitance in the transistors and in other components of the amplifiers. In conventional neurodiagnostic equipment, the draw of current from the signal voltage source and from the preceding amplifier stage is many orders of magnitude less than the output current and therefore negligible.

Differential Amplifiers

The *differential amplifier*, sometimes called a "balanced amplifier," is used extensively in neurophysiologic equipment. Its major advantage is the property of *common mode rejection*. A standard amplifier compares a signal voltage in the active input to a common reference (Figure 4.5A). Un-

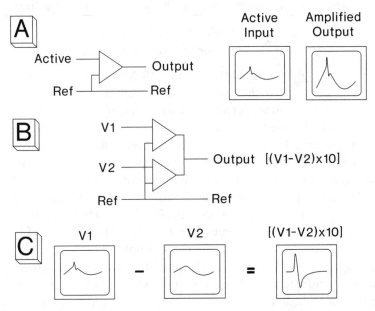

Figure 4.5 Single-ended and differential amplifiers. *(A)* Single-ended amplifier. The output is a magnified representation of the input. *(B)* Differential amplifier. The output is a magnified representation of the difference between the two signals, V_1 and V_2. *(C)* Simulated oscilloscope traces of the inputs and output of the differential amplifier shown in B. The slow activity in common to both inputs is magnified equally but cancels out because the second channel output is inverted. The spike, which is only seen in V_1, is amplified in the output.

wanted signals are amplified the same as biological signals. The main un-wanted signal in clinical situations is 60-Hz activity (line voltage through nearby electrical circuits).

The differential amplifier is designed to reject unwanted signals through the use of an inverting circuit. The power supply voltage is inverted, so that a positive input voltage results in a proportional negative output voltage. In all other respects it functions as a standard amplifier. In Figure 4.5B, the signal voltages V_1 and V_2 are compared. The standard amplifier is labeled "+10×," whereas the inverting amplifier is "–10×." The output voltage is the sum of the two amplifiers.

The effect of this arrangement is that any signal applied in common to the two electrodes (V_1 and V_2) cancel each other out and are not seen in the output (that is, the modes in common to the two electrodes are rejected, or common mode rejection). The 60-Hz activity affects both inputs equally and is canceled out; the result is an improved output signal (Figure 4.5C).

The common mode rejection does not work as well on high-amplitude signals because the input impedance and the amplifying characteristics of the two amplifiers are not exactly the same. The common mode rejection ratio (CMRR) is equal to applied common input voltage divided by the output voltage.

$$CMRR = \frac{\text{Common signal voltage}}{\text{Nonamplified output voltage}}$$

For modern amplifiers the CMRR is about 10,000 to 1. However, the CMRR can be degraded by very high or very different electrode impedances that serve to change the signal voltage perceived by the inputs of the amplifiers.

The differential amplifier is used for EEGs in montages that compare two electrodes. In Figure 4.6, the preamplifiers first boost the signal for ease of filtering and noise reduction and then feed the amplified signals to the amplifiers. In this diagram, the standard and the inverting amplifiers are included in one amplifier symbol (the V_2 for one channel is the V_1 for the next). This is an example of the left parasaggital portion of the longitudinal bipolar (LB) montage.

This serial bipolar arrangement is responsible for the reversal of localized cortical potentials. Using Figure 4.6 as an example, consider the display of a surface negative spike focus at C3. The amplifier arrangement would deliver a negative potential to the top input of a differential amplifier, causing an upward pen deflection, and a negative potential to the bottom input, causing a downward pen deflection. The signal produced by a negative potential at C3 is seen predominantly in two channels: F3-C3 and C3-P3. In the F3-C3 channel, the negative spike in the bottom input to the differential amplifier causes a downward pen deflection and the negative potential in the top input of the C3-P3 of the differential amplifier causes an upward pen deflection. Therefore, the two spikes point toward each other (toward the focus) when the two channels are displayed serially on paper.

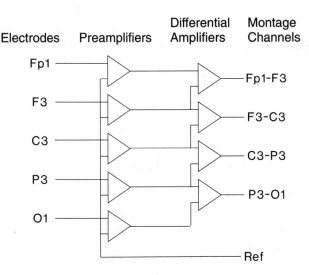

Figure 4.6 EEG amplifier. Preamplifiers boost signal intensity and feed their output to the differential amplifiers. In this figure, the differential amplifiers are represented as a single symbol. The electrodes and connections comprise the left parasaggital portion of the longitudinal bipolar montage. Note that in this bipolar montage, the secondary (inverted) input for one channel is the primary (noninverted) signal for the next.

Signal Averaging

Averaging is needed for neurodiagnostic studies that require the identification of small amplitude potentials (that is, evoked potentials and sensory nerve action potentials). The steps to averaging are as follows:

1. Recording of analog signals
2. Digitization of the signal
3. Storage of the data points into memory
4. Acquisition and digitization of additional trials with addition of data points in memory
5. Division of data registers by the number of trials
6. Display of the averaged waveform.

Analog-to-Digital Conversion

An analog signal is a wave that fluctuates continuously in voltage. Digital conversion consists of measuring the voltage at regular intervals and recording the voltage into a region of computer memory (Figure 4.7). Computers store information in digital format, so the analog voltage at each specified time is converted into a binary format by dividing the voltage range into several levels coded in binary format. For example, with a two-bit A/D converter, the possible combinations of the two bits are:

Binary	Decimal
00	0
01	1
10	2
11	3

With a three-bit converter, the possibilities are:

Binary	Decimal
000	0
001	1
010	2
011	3
100	4
101	5
110	6
111	7

Therefore, the number of possible levels is equal to 2 raised to the power of the number of bits. $2^2 = 4$, $2^3 = 8$. Since most neurodiagnostic equipment uses A/D converters of at least twelve bits, $2^{12} = 4096$. Four thousand voltage levels is more than sufficient to accurately represent any physiological analog signal.

Time resolution of the A/D converter depends on capabilities of the converter, duration of the recording epoch, and number of channels to be sampled. Speed of conversion can be described by at least three terms: sampling rate, intersample interval (ISI), and dwell time. *Sampling rate* is preferred; it simply indicates the number of conversions per second. *ISI* is the inverse of sampling rate, and is expressed as ms or μs. *Dwell time* is similar to ISI, but should probably not be used. It is misleading in that one might conceive of the A/D converter "dwelling" on the sample for the entire time, perhaps continuously sampling during that interval. In reality, the converter takes its sample, then waits until the internal clock says it is time to take the next sample.

Most A/D converters can convert at least 40,000 samples per second. Many do much better. An A/D converter can sample several channels; however, it must do it sequentially: for example, channel 1, then channel 2, then channel 3, then channel 4, then back to channel 1. In this example, the maximum conversion rate per channel would be 40,000/4 or 10,000 samples per second. Clearly, the more channels sampled, the poorer the time resolution of the averaged signal. Epoch duration determines how many samples will be needed. The sampling rate must be set to be appropriate to the epoch duration. For example, if you want to sample an epoch of 10 seconds for a sympathetic skin response, sampling at 100,000 per second would be excessive. Not only is that

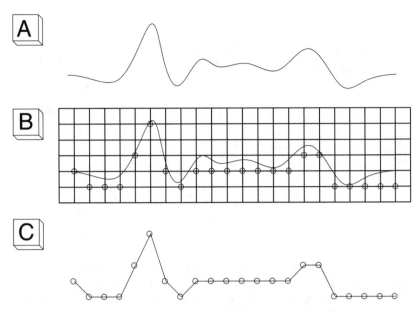

Figure 4.7   Analog to digital conversion. *(A)* Analog biologic signal that is to be digitized. *(B)* Grid is placed over the signal. Each vertical line is the time of sampling. Each horizontal line is a voltage level that can be discerned by the digital converter. At each sampling time, the highest voltage level crossed is the digital voltage recorded. A dot at the intersection of the time and voltage line indicates the digitally measured data point. *(C)* Waveform reconstructed from the digitized data. The wave is essentially lines connecting the digitized data points.

degree of resolution not necessary, but the computer memory would probably not be able to handle the 1,000,000 data points.

On the other hand, sampling at too slow a rate degrades the recording. *Aliasing* refers to an error that occurs when the sampling rate is too slow for the frequency components of the signal. Figure 4.8 illustrates this. *A* shows the simulated biological signal that is a sine wave. The vertical lines are the sampling times. The dots are the voltages measured at each sampling time. *B* is the waveform reconstructed from the data points measured in *A*. The wave has a sine-like appearance; however, the frequency of the wave is much lower than that of the original signal. In order to adequately represent a digitized frequency, the sampling rate must be at least twice the frequency of the fastest component.

Averaging

Signal averaging consists of acquisition of multiple trials, digitization of each trial, and averaging of the digital data in the computer's memory. The first trial is stored directly in the computer's memory. Subse-

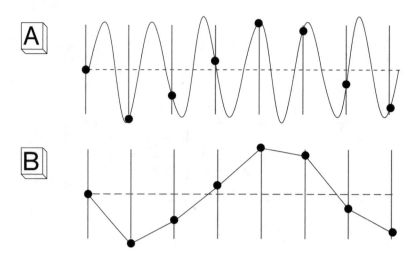

Figure 4.8 Aliasing. *(A)* Sine-wave signal. Vertical lines are sampling times of the A/D converter. Dots are measured voltages at each sampling time. *(B)* Waveform reconstructed using the data points measured in *A*. The frequency of this wave is much less than that of the original signal.

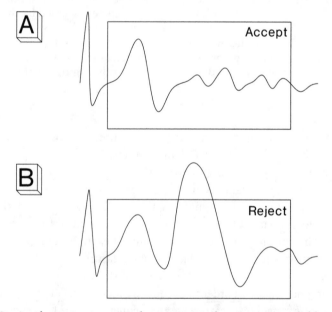

Figure 4.9 Artifact rejection. An electronic window is represented by vertical lines. *(A)* The potential falls completely within the window. Therefore, this trace will be accepted into the average. The stimulus artifact at the beginning of the trace occurs before the sampling begins; therefore, this does not prevent acceptance of the trial. *(B)* A high-voltage transient falls outside of the window. The entire trace will be rejected. Depending on software, the display will indicate Accept or Reject on the display or separate indicator.

quently, each additional trial is recorded in memory and the total divided by the number of acquired trials. In this way, the computer memory holds a running average of the trials.

Artifact Rejection

Artifact rejection is an essential part of every signal averaging program (see Figure 4.9). The averager rejects from the average any trial that appears contaminated by artifact. An electronic window is preset so that the averager can distinguish artifact from physiological signals. The entire trial is rejected if it contains any potentials whose amplitude is outside the window, because high-voltage inputs to an amplifier may produce a temporary block of the amplifier response, which would cause instability of amplification and frequency response for several seconds.

5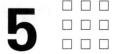

Displays

Displays are basically one of two types: paper or cathode-ray tube (CRT). Both display changes in signal with time.

Paper Display

Electroencephalographic (EEG) recording is usually accomplished by the movement of paper past pens whose vertical movements are governed by the amplified signal. After passage through filters and preamplifiers, the signal voltage is fed to a driver amplifier. The output is connected to a resistor and coil attached to the pen (Figure 5.1, resistor not shown). The pen coil, in turn, is mounted between poles of a permanent magnet. The passage of an amplified signal current through the coil produces a magnetic field that is oriented so that it acts on the permanent magnetic field to deflect the pen. Most of the time, a spring keeps the pen pointing in the right direction, but the fluctuating electromagnetic field moves the pen from this center position. Some pen arrangements use counterbalancing electromagnets to control pen position rather than a single electromagnet and spring. Others use slightly different arrangements, but, in all of these, the basic mechanism is as described here.

Two important properties of EEG recording pens are inertia and nonlinearity. Inertia is caused by their weight; more torque is required to get the pen moving than to keep it moving, resulting in the pen's tendency to overshoot when made to move rapidly. Overshoot is compensated for by electrical and mechanical damping. Electrical damping is accomplished by a feedback circuit to the pen driver amplifier that corrects the pen position when it overshoots its target position. Mechanical damping is accomplished by varying pen pressure. Damping is not perfect, and alterations in damping change the frequency response of the record.

Nonlinearity is largely due to the pivot mechanism that produces an arc rather than a straight vertical line (see right side of Figure 5.1). Since the signal voltage proportionately determines pen angle, the relationship between signal voltage and vertical distance from baseline to pen tip is not linear.

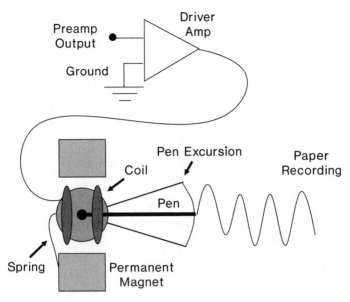

Figure 5.1   Paper display. Output from the driver amplifier is delivered to a coil attached to the pen. Current passing through the coil creates a magnetic field that makes the pen pivot within the field of the permanent magnets.

Cathode-ray Tube

Evoked potential (EP) and electromyographic (EMG) equipment use CRTs, which have the ability to display much faster signal changes than the pen display of EEG. This is because the projected electrons have little mass or inertia. The pen, on the other hand, has substantial inertia, by virtue of the coil, pivot mechanism, and pen itself.

The CRT uses a controlled beam of electrons (the cathode ray) to excite phosphors on the screen for visible display (Figure 5.2). The source of the electrons is a hot cathode; a large amount of energy is imparted to the electrons so that they can escape the parent metal. The electrons are accelerated and focused into a beam by a series of plate electrodes, chiefly anodes (that attract electrons). After the beam is focused, it passes between two sets of deflecting plates oriented at right angles to each other. The deflecting plates control the horizontal and vertical movement of the beam. For EMG and EP, the amplified signal voltage is applied across the plates controlling vertical movements, and a time base signal controls the horizontal movements. The time base is a ramp voltage delivered to the horizontal deflecting plates that causes the beam to move gradually from left to right with time. At the completion of the sweep, the horizontal plate voltage quickly changes back so that the beam is ready to make another sweep. The time base refers to the speed of the horizontal ramp voltage and, therefore, to the speed of movement of the beam on the

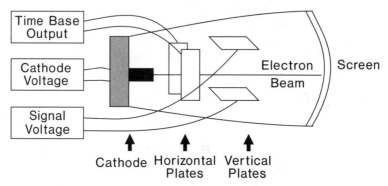

Figure 5.2   Cathode-ray tube. A hot cathode creates an electron source that is accelerated and focused by the anode. Output from the time base is delivered to the plates governing horizontal deflection of the electron beam. Output from the driver amplifier is delivered to the plates governing vertical deflection of the electron beam. Impact of the electron beam onto the screen causes phosphorescence and emission of photons.

screen. Figure 5.3A illustrates the actions of different time base settings on the voltage applied to the horizontal deflecting plates of the CRT.

The sweep can be triggered in several ways, as in Figure 5.3B. In EMG needle studies, the sweep begins as soon as the previous sweep is completed. In stimulus-triggered sweeps, the time base begins the horizontal ramp when it receives a pulse from the stimulator. Line triggering is more complicated. In this case, the sweep is triggered when a signal of sufficient amplitude and rise time is received along the biological signal channel. This type of triggering is used to examine jitter on EMG.

On the CRT, electrons transfer energy upon impact into the phosphor. As energy is lost, photons of light are emitted from the phosphor for visual display.

When studying nerve-conduction velocity (NCV), the amplification is chosen so that the takeoff and peak of the signal are easily measured, and the time base is selected so that the waves of interest are displayed farthest apart while still on the same sweep speed. Error is introduced when the time base is too slow or is changed between proximal and distal stimuli.

The gain used in the EMG needle study must vary so that the waves of interest are displayed optimally on the screen. The amplitude of waveforms varies from 50 μV/divisions (div) for spontaneous activity to 1 to 2 mV/div for maximal motor unit activation. The time base chosen is the fastest at which individual sweeps can be clearly delineated. When sweep speeds are faster than 16 frames/sec, one cannot determine whether two waves are on the same sweep or on subsequent sweeps. This is termed the *flicker-fusion frequency*. At 10 ms/div, the distinction between sweeps is easily made. Since there are ten divisions on a screen, that is a sweep time of 100 ms, or a frequency of 10 sweeps/sec. If 5 ms/div is used, then each sweep takes 50 ms, or a frequency of 20 sweeps/sec, that is, faster than the flicker-fusion frequency.

Evoked responses are displayed on CRTs, although data handling is substantially different from EMGs. This is discussed in detail in Part IV. Evoked Potentials.

Other Methods

Most paper displays continue to use standard pens. Some machines, however, use a dot-matrix print head, sometimes using jets of ink. The quality of these recordings is good, although close inspection can easily detect the composite nature. These print heads avoid two major pitfalls of mechanical pens, inertia and arc effect from the swinging pen.

Ink can be sprayed onto paper in a number of ways, most commonly by heat. The print head contains many small holes. Behind the holes is a thin layer of ink in continuity with a reservoir. Behind the ink is a plate containing tiny heating elements. A command from a microprocessor tells the heating element to become hot quickly. A bubble forms as the temperature soars almost instantaneously. The bubble expands, displacing ink. The force of the expansion results in sufficient pressure to spray ink through the hole and onto the paper. The element then cools, allowing the bubble to collapse. As the bubble collapses, the area behind the opening fills with ink from the reservoir. This is the basic idea behind "ink jet" or "bubble-jet" printers.

Thermal-transfer printers use heat to produce an imprint on special paper. The heat evokes a color change on the paper. Thermal transfer is used by some strip-chart printers, such as on EMG and EKG machines.

6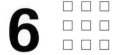

✓ Electrodes and the Patient-Electrode Interface

All neurophysiologic equipment requires electrodes. It is a common misconception that the electrodes pick up the electrical activity and the equipment records it. Rather, the electrodes make the patient an integral part of the circuitry of the equipment. The rest of the circuit is designed to record the amount of current flow in the loop formed by the patient, electrodes, and input circuits of the amplifiers. Therefore, the important features in understanding neurodiagnostic equipment are the electrodes, the electrode/patient interface, and the electrode/amplifier interface.

Electrode Theory

The recorded electrical activity is generated by charge movement in brain, muscle, or nerve. The charge movement is conducted into one electrode, through the circuitry of the amplifier, and back into the patient through another electrode. Therefore, the patient and amplifier form a complete circuit loop. The electrodes allow this charge transfer.

Electroencephalographic Electrodes

Inserting electroencephalographic (EEG) and evoked potential (EP) electrodes into conducting gel is more complex than it seems. Abrasion of the skin is done largely to remove oils and layers of dead skin that contain low levels of electrolytes for conduction. Electrolyte gel then connects the skin and electrode. The gel is essentially a malleable extension of the electrode; it maximizes skin contact and is required for low-resistance recording through the skin.

gel ↓ resistance through the skin.

Electrodes may be reversible or nonreversible. The nonreversible nature of some electrodes is due to polarization of the junction between the gel and electrode, which reduces current flow through the junction. Essentially, the junction has features of a diode and a capacitor. Current flows in only one direction, which results in the charging of the capacitance with no ability to discharge. In this situation, little current will flow and signal will be lost, especially at lower frequencies, since these have greater potential to charge the capacitance. Reversible electrodes allow for charge to pass through the junction in both directions, although these also have small junction potentials. An electrode is reversible because either (1) the electrode has ions in common with the gel, or (2) the electrode and gel contain dissimilar ions at two valence states, allowing for mutual oxidation/reduction reactions to transfer charge.

The best-known electrode-gel system is a chlorided silver (AgCl) electrode in a sodium chloride (NaCl) solution. Before using the electrodes, silver (Ag) electrodes must first be oxidized using chloride. To do this, the electrode is placed in a NaCl solution and electric current passed through the electrode into the solution. In the solution, the NaCl dissociates into Na^+ and Cl^-. The Cl^- binds to the Ag to form AgCl on the electrode. The current is required to impart a positive charge to the silver so it will accept the Cl^-. Formulae for this process are as follows:

$$NaCl = Na^+ + Cl^- \qquad \text{(in water)}$$

$$Ag = Ag^+ + e^- \qquad \text{(in the electrode)}$$

$$Ag^+ + Cl^- = AgCl \qquad \text{(at electrode surface)}$$

$$Na^+ + e^- + H_2O = NaOH + \tfrac{1}{2}(H_2) \qquad \text{(to clean up)}$$

Once the electrode has been chlorided, it is placed in a gel that contains Cl^- ions, such as NaCl, as above. Then, conduction of charge across the junction is similar to the chloriding process in forward and reverse.

Figure 6.1A is a schematic diagram of the ionic fluxes during the recording of an EEG signal. A negative charge arises from the head forcing Cl^- from the skin into the gel. Subsequently, the Cl^- combines with Ag^+ to give AgCl and a free electron (e–). This travels to the amplifier to complete the flow of charge.

The functions of the skin/gel/electrode interfaces are complex, but can largely be modeled by the use of circuit elements (Figure 6.1B). In this diagram, Rs is the resistance of the gel; C is the capacitance of the interface; Rf is the resistance of the chemical reaction that moves charge at the interface; W is the "Warburg impedance," which is a frequency-dependent resistance; and Co

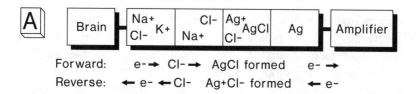

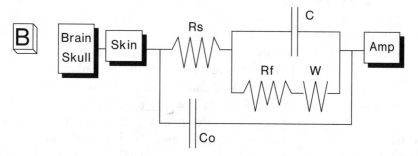

Figure 6.1 Interface between patient and machine. *(A)* Ionic fluxes during the recording of EEG signals. *(B)* Circuit simulating the interface among skin, gel, and electrode.

is an additional element of capacitance that, in reality, is too small to be of major importance. The most important part of the circuit is the central loop made by C, Rf, and W. In a reversible surface electrode the capacitance (C) is fairly large and the resistance of Rf and W are small. Thus, there is little modification of the incoming signal, since the capacitor is essentially bypassed for low frequencies, and higher frequencies may be conducted through both arms of the circuit. However, with a nonreversible electrode, the resistances through Rf and W are large; therefore, current flows onto the capacitor, resulting in a buildup of charge. This essentially acts like a low-frequency filter, blocking the transmission of low frequencies to the amplifier. Therefore, nonreversible electrodes are not satisfactory for recording EEG.

Electromyographic Electrodes

The design and function of needle electrodes is fairly easy to conceptualize. The needle electrode is inserted into the muscle, where electrical activity of the muscle fibers is detected. The voltage changes of nearby fibers cause a very small amount of current to flow through a coaxial electrode and through its leads to the amplifier before completing the circuit through the reference electrode and tissue. Although the electrode impedance is fairly small, the amplifier input impedance is large, so the actual amount of current flowing into the amplifier is small.

Electrode-Amplifier Interface

When several amplifiers are connected in series, each amplifier draws little current from the preceding amplifier. This is also true of the interface between the amplifiers and the electrode connected to the signal source. In the case of EEG and EMG, electrode resistances are kept relatively low for two reasons: (1) to decrease electrical noise, and (2) to make the recorded potential a true representation of the physiological potential. Noise will be discussed in chapter 7.

The relationship between electrode resistance and amplifier input resistance is as important as the absolute resistances. We can consider the connection of an electrode to the biological signal source to be an electrical circuit, in Figure 6.2A, with the electrode resistance (Re) and amplifier input resistance (Rin) being in series with the signal voltage (Vs).

Current *(I)* flows around the circuit, and from Ohm's law:

$$Vs = I \times Req \tag{6.1}$$

and

$$Vs = Ve + Vin \tag{6.2}$$

and also

$$Ve = I \times Re \text{ and } Vin = I \times Rin \tag{6.3}$$

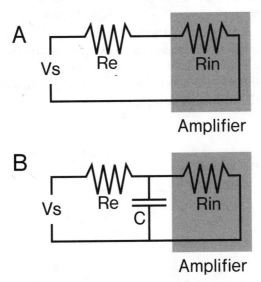

Figure 6.2 Electrode-amplifier interface. *(A)* Simple circuit created by the electrode and amplifier. *(B)* Circuit of electrode and amplifier with capacitance represented by the capacitor symbol. This is not a manufactured capacitor, but rather capacitance among electrode leads, tissues, and equipment.

where Ve is the voltage drop across the electrode and Vin is the voltage drop across the amplifier input resistance. Remember that Vin is what will be amplified. Dividing equation (6.2) by Vs and rearranging we get:

$$\frac{Vin}{Vs} = \frac{Vs - Ve}{Vs}$$

Now substituting in equation (6.3):

$$\frac{Vin}{Vs} = \frac{(I \times Req) - (I \times Re)}{(I \times Req)}$$

where $Req = Re + Rin$. So:

$$\frac{Vin}{Vs} = \frac{Rin}{(Re + Rin)}$$

This equation means that the ratio of the amplifier input voltage to the signal voltage approaches 1 only when the input resistance of the amplifier (Rin) is much greater than the electrode resistance (Re). In general, the input resistance is kept at least two orders of magnitude (100x) greater than the electrode resistance, so that the input voltage is at least 99% of the signal voltage.

We have been referring to the electrode and amplifier input resistance; however, remember that they are actually impedances, since impedance is frequency-dependent resistance. This implies that there must be an element of capacitance in the circuit even though we have not drawn it in the previous diagrams (see Figure 6.2B). The capacitances come from the tissue, connecting wires, and other components of the electrical circuits. The equations for impedance would result in the same basic conceptual conclusions, but the mathematics would be much more complex.

7

□ □ □
□ □ □
□ □ □

√Artifacts and Noise

Signal-to-Noise Ratio

A recording is composed of signal plus noise. What is signal and what is noise depends on what you are measuring. For example, in conventional electroencephalography (EEG), the signal-to-noise (S/N) ratio is high, meaning that with good technique the signal is clearly discernible from other electrical activity. In contrast, for evoked potentials, not only is the response much smaller in amplitude, but the normal EEG background is part of the noise, obscuring the recording. Therefore, a signal-to-noise ratio is defined for the signal under study only after filtering. The signal-to-noise ratio is usually calculated from absolute amplitude. *Absolute* means that the signal is rectified for calculation, that is, all negative values are made positive. Signal-to-noise ratio can also be expressed in terms of power.

The best ways to maximize signal-to-noise ratio are:

- Good technique
- Preamplifier in the head stage
- Averaging.

Some important features of technique include (1) equal electrode impedances, so there is no degradation of common mode rejection, (2) short electrode leads and power cords to avoid stray capacitance and inductance, and (3) proper grounding and selection of location for equipment to minimize electrical noise.

A preamplifier in the head stage of the equipment magnifies the signal so that it is not as susceptible to degradation by electrical interference. The effect of stray capacitance is proportionately less on a 10-mV signal than a 1-mV signal.

Averaging is the only way to improve the signal-to-noise ratio of evoked potentials, and is helpful for sensory nerve action potentials. The signal-to-noise ratio improves with increasing number of averaged trials. If the ratio is expressed in terms of amplitude, the ratio improves by a factor of the square root of the number of samples.

Averaged signal S/N ratio = Single sample S/N ratio × *√N

where N is the number of samples.

If the ratio is expressed in terms of power, the ratio improves in proportion to the number of samples. The following lists some sample signal-to-noise ratios (as amplitude) for numbers of samples:

Samples	Improvement in S/N ratio
2	1.4
4	2.0
8	2.8
16	4.0
100	10.0
1,000	31.6
2,000	44.7
10,000	100.0

The signal-to-noise ratio is the best index of clarity of recording. In general, avoiding the sources of artifacts described in the next section will improve the signal-to-noise ratio.

There are many potential sources of artifacts and noise in neurodiagnostic recordings. Only the basic principles will be discussed in this text.

60-Hertz Noise

Two of the most important factors causing electrical noise are stray capacitance and stray inductance. The small amount of capacitance that exists among electrode wires, power lines, and tissue-gel-electrode interface allows a charge gradient to be built up (called *stray capacitance*). The charge can flow in an unpredictable manner into the amplifier or alter the response of the amplifier to the physiological potential. Since the stray capacitance is variable and the charge movement is influenced by signal voltages or line voltages, for example, the effect is virtually impossible to predict and is seen as noise.

Stray inductance is the production of current in a wire by a surrounding magnetic field. For example, the movement of current through the wires of a light will produce a weak magnetic field. This magnetic field can induce electrons to flow in another wire, such as an electrode lead. This effect is negligible if electrode resistances are small and the signal current flow is large. However, if electrode resistances are high and the signal current flow is small, then induced current becomes a substantial fraction of the total current input to the amplifier. This is one reason why 60-Hz interference is more prominent when electrodes have high impedances (for example, a broken wire, a loose electrode lead, or an electrode with normally high impedance such as a microelectrode).

Common mode rejection was previously mentioned as one of the most important features of EEG machines responsible for eliminating 60-Hz noise (see chapter 4 on amplifiers). This effect is degraded by high or unequal electrode impedances, loss of proper ground, or smear of electrode gel between the ground and an active electrode. Electrode gel smear is not detected by insuring that electrode impedances are less than 5 kohms.

In summary, the measures that reduce 60-Hz activity are (1) insuring proper ground, (2) keeping electrode impedances that are relatively low and approximately equal, (3) using reversible electrodes, (4) keeping power lines away from electrode leads, and (5) electrical shielding of room and/or cables. In addition to these measures, some equipment uses additional electronic techniques to reduce noise.

Movement Artifact

Movement of the patient or the electrode wires during EEG or EMG recordings results in relatively high amplitude artifacts, caused by a disturbance in the junction potentials between electrode and gel or gel and skin, and by movement of electrode leads.

Junction potentials are stable only as long as the electrode system is stationary. Movement disturbs the ionic gradients that have developed and causes charge to move down potential gradients. The input to the amplifier changes because the capacitance of the system had previously negated the effect of the junction potentials (that is, the direct current [DC] shift was essentially filtered out). With time, the junction potential reforms. This process can also be perceived by the input amplifier as a slow electrical potential change. Moving electrode leads changes the amount of stray capacitance and changes the distribution of current caused by stray inductance.

[handwritten: don't high Elect. impedance & loose electrodes] *[handwritten: only common to one Electrode & ground but seen in all channels having that electrode]*

Electrode Pops

Electrode pops are spike-like potentials that occur in an apparently random fashion and are caused by sudden changes in junction potentials. A high junction potential and the junction of dissimilar metals are conditions predisposed to electrode pops. An imperceptible movement or alteration in electrode-gel interface can temporarily short out the junction potential. This sudden change in DC potential delivered to the amplifier is seen in all channels with that electrode in common. As the stable junction potential is reestablished, the amplifier (and pen deflection) returns to baseline. Dissimilar metals build up large junction potentials that are subsequently discharged into the input amplifier. The discharge can cycle repetitively at irregular rates, depending on electrode and wire movement and ongoing electrocerebral activity. High electrode impedances and loose electrodes also predispose to electrode pops.

8

□ □ □
□ □ □
□ □ □

Electrical Safety

The principles of electrical safety are intended to protect the patient from potentially lethal currents while optimal recording of biological signals is obtained. Line power in a hospital is supplied by three wires; the hot lead has black insulation, the neutral has white insulation, and the ground has green insulation or is an uninsulated (usually copper) wire. The hot line carries an alternating ±110 V. The neutral is the ground reference from the power company. Its voltage may not be exactly at zero. The ground is the building ground connection.

The chief concern in electrical safety is leakage current. Leakage current has several sources; two of these, stray capacitance and stray inductance, are often easily detected because they also accentuate electrical noise. When dealing with leakage current, the capacitance and inductance are mainly in the power supply wires. This condition can increase the potential differences of references and grounds to much greater than zero volts. The amount of leakage current depends on the length and capacitance of the wires. Therefore, extension cords should not be used during electrophysiological recordings. For example, a six-foot-long power cord may produce up to 70 µA of leak current. Figure 8.1 shows a diagram of a patient hooked up to a machine *(A)* and an equivalent electrical circuit diagram of this situation *(B)*.

The delivery of leak currents to patients is increased when a ground fault exists. This usually occurs when the ground connection of a piece of equipment is lost. The most common causes are either a broken ground wire in the power cord or loss of building ground. If the power cord wire is broken, repair is always made since the machine does not work; however, the operator may not know if the ground connection is broken without specifically testing it. With the loss of building ground, especially in older buildings where the third wire was added later, some electricians install a three-prong plug to the wall but attach the ground connection to the plug box, which has only a weak connection or no connection at all to earth ground. The deleterious effect of these conditions is enhanced if a patient is attached to two pieces of electrical equipment where one is adequately grounded and the other is not. If the patient is

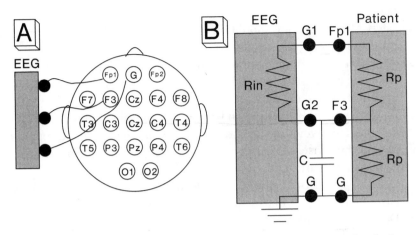

Figure 8.1 Patient-equipment interface. *(A)* Diagram of a patient hooked up to an EEG machine. The cartoon of the head is a standard diagram for indicating electrode positions. Electrode placement follows the 10-20 Electrode Placement System (see part II). The electrode connections shown are for the first channel of the longitudinal bipolar montage. *(B)* Equivalent electric circuit to some of the connections in A. The capacitor (C) represents the capacitance of the electrode leads and equipment; it is not a true capacitor.

grounded to both pieces, then leak current can flow from the ground wire of one machine, through the patient, and into the ground of the other machine. The practical extension of this example is that only one ground should be attached to a patient, and all equipment attached to a patient should be connected to the same power strip and to a single ground.

Ground loops also degrade the recording of the biological signal, since they introduce the potential for greatly magnified 60-Hz interference. Basically, the loop acts like a transformer coil, that is, magnetic fields in the environment cause relatively large amounts of current to flow in the wires. Current has the potential to flow through the patient as part of this loop. The loop can be minimized by using the same outlets for all of the interconnected equipment and making sure that only one ground is used on the patient.

Leakage current poses the greatest threat to patients when it is applied directly to the myocardium, which is possible in patients with a temporary pacemaker. Patients can be classified into three categories of electrical risk according to the amount of current that is safely applied: (1) patients not connected to electrical equipment = 500 μamp; (2) patients connected by surface electrodes to electrical apparatus (for example, EKG or EEG monitors) = 100 μamp; and (3) patients with a direct conductive pathway to the heart = 10 μamp. The following is a suggested set of guidelines for electrical safety:

1. Electrical equipment for patient use must be inspected regularly for

safety. The inspection should include verification of proper ground and measurement of leakage current.

2. All electrical equipment attached to a patient should be plugged into the same power strip to avoid ground loops and to minimize the possibility of ground faults.

3. Machines should be turned on before attaching electrodes to the patient. This avoids power surges that may be transmitted through the patient. Likewise, the patient should be disconnected before the equipment is turned off.

4. Use only one patient ground. This decreases the opportunity for leak currents from other machinery to pass through the patient.

5. Do not use extension cords, in order to avoid increasing leakage currents.

6. When recording electromyographs, be sure the ground is on the same limb as the active electrode so that leakage currents do not flow through the heart.

Electroencephalography

9

Physiological Basis of Electroencephalography

[handwritten] EEG activity recorded at scalp is generated
← Source of the activity by the action potentials of cortical neurons
← but most is generated by EPSP and IPSP.

Electroencephalography (EEG) is the recording of brain electrical activity. Some of the activity recorded by scalp electrodes is generated by action potentials of cortical neurons but most is generated by excitatory postsynaptic potentials (EPSP) and inhibitory postsynaptic potentials (IPSP).

Basic Neurophysiology

Neural transmission occurs by sequential depolarization and repolarization of neural membranes. Depolarization of the nerve terminal causes release of transmitter into the synaptic cleft. The action of transmitter on the postsynaptic membrane causes a change in conductance to certain ions, which in turn results in either depolarization or hyperpolarization of the cell. Depolarization is usually excitatory while hyperpolarization is inhibitory. Most neurons use action potentials to propagate activity over long distances. In contrast, many interneurons do not generate action potentials; rather, depolarization of postsynaptic membrane causes depolarization of the adjacent membrane. If the release site is depolarized sufficiently, transmitter is released onto the next cell. This is termed *electrotonic conduction* (illustrated in Figure 9.1).

[handwritten] → Propagated action potential
neuron → electrotonic dc conduction

Action Potentials

[handwritten] neuron, outer neuron

Action potentials are generated in the axon hillock when the amount of depolarization is sufficient to reach threshold. Depolarization of the membrane opens voltage-dependent sodium channels that allow the influx of sodium. This influx depolarizes the cell beyond zero potential and a small positive potential is generated. The action potential is terminated by closure of the sodium channels. These channels are not only voltage dependent, but also time dependent. The channels close at the end of a specified time and then cannot be

[handwritten] Na+ channels are not only voltage dependent but also time dependent
(1 msec)

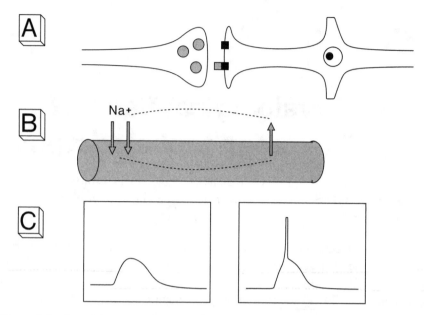

Figure 9.1 Synaptic transmission and action potentials. *(A)* Basic mechanisms of synaptic transmission. Depolarization of the terminal on the left causes release of transmitter vesicles (hatched circles) into the cleft. The transmitter (hatched box) binds to the postsynaptic receptor (solid box). *(B)* Electrotonic depolarization of adjacent membrane. Inward current on the left results in depolarization of membrane further to the right. *(C)* Effect of depolarization on membrane potential. Left is a potential that does not reach threshold. Right is a potential that reaches threshold and results in an action potential. Threshold is indicated by the dashed line.

reopened until the membrane has repolarized. Closure of the sodium channels allows potassium diffusion to reestablish the resting potential.

Synaptic Transmission

Synaptic transmission occurs with the release of neuro–transmitter from the presynaptic terminal onto the postsynaptic terminal. Depolarization of the presynaptic terminal causes an influx of calcium. Calcium facilitates fusion of vesicles with the terminal membrane, thereby releasing transmitter into the cleft. The transmitter diffuses across the cleft and binds to receptors on the postsynaptic membrane. This binding causes opening of specific ionic channels. The nature of the ionic movements determines whether the postsynaptic potential is excitatory or inhibitory.

Excitatory Postsynaptic Potentials
↑ conductance to Na^+ & Ca^{++} ions

Excitatory synaptic transmission is caused by depolarization of the cell toward threshold. Excitatory postsynaptic potentials (EPSPs) usually occur due to an increased conductance to sodium and/or calcium. As the conductance to sodium increases, the influx diminishes the resting membrane potential so that the cell approaches zero potential. Because the conductance to sodium is greater than to any other ion, the membrane potential approaches the equilibrium potential for sodium, which is positive (approximately +45 mV).

Several EPSPs may be needed to generate sufficient depolarization to produce a regenerative action potential. Therefore, the release of transmitter is dependent on action potential generation, and is therefore "all-or-none." Some interneurons do not generate action potentials. Instead, depolarization of the postsynaptic membrane is electrotonically conducted to the cell's own terminal. This depolarization in turn produces release of transmitter. Since the release of transmitter is directly related to the degree of depolarization, the transmission is graded, rather than all-or-none, as for action-potential-generating neurons.

Inhibitory Postsynaptic Potentials
↑ conductance to K^+ or cl^- ions

Inhibitory synaptic transmission is caused by increased conductance to potassium and/or chloride. The equilibrium potential for potassium is more negative than the resting membrane potential, so increased potassium conductance hyperpolarizes the cell. The equilibrium potential for chloride is more positive than the resting membrane potential but still negative, approximately –55 mV. Therefore, increased conductance to chloride depolarizes the membrane but effectively clamps the membrane potential from becoming much less than –55 mV.

Generation of Electroencephalographic Rhythms

Scalp electrodes detect charge movement only in the most superficial regions of the cerebral cortex. Electrical activity in the deep nuclei produces surface potentials of very low amplitude. These potentials are overwhelmed by cortical activity. Therefore, a discussion of generation of EEG rhythms must concentrate on generation of cortical potentials.

Cortical Potentials

The cerebral cortex functions in a manner similar to most nuclei. The cortex receives input, processing is facilitated by interneurons, and output is projected to other regions (Figure 9.2). Throughout most of the cor-

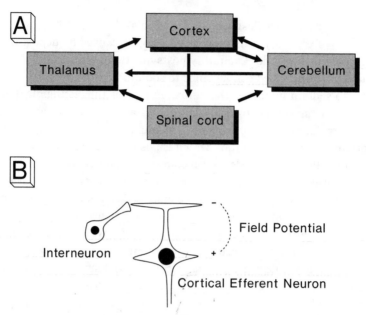

Figure 9.2 Cortical and subcortical organization. *(A)* Efferent neurons have projections to subcortical structures as well as intracortical projections (not shown). Afferent input to the cortex comes from both deep cerebral nuclei plus ascending afferents from the brainstem and spinal cord. *(B)* Close-up of the cortex showing synapse of an excitatory interneuron on the dendrites of a cortical efferent neuron. Depolarization of superficial dendrites results in a negative field potential in the upper layers of the cortex. Electrotonic depolarization of the soma and axon hillock results in a positive field potential in deeper layers.

tex, the largest neurons are the source of efferent outflow. These neurons are oriented perpendicular to the cortical surface, such that dendritic arborizations are prominent in superficial layers and the soma and axon hillock are located in deeper layers. This creates a vertical columnar organization of the cortex.

Activation of thalamocortical afferents results in EPSPs and IPSPs in the interneurons and efferent neurons. Depolarization of the dendrites is conducted along the cell membrane to the axon hillock, where an efferent action potential is generated. Efferent action potentials project to nuclei in the subcortex, brainstem, spinal cord, and other cortical regions. The influx of positive ions into the efferent neuron results in a negative extracellular field potential. Electrotonic depolarization of the soma and axon hillock results in a positive field potential. Because of the vertical organization of the large efferent neurons, the negative field potential is usually superficial to the positive field potential. This is a dipole. While the term *dipole* is usually used to describe the orientation of epileptiform activity, virtually all electrophysiologic potentials can be represented, at least in theory, as a positive/negative dipole.

[handwritten: the afferent generator for the occipital alpha rythm is thought to be the thalamus.]

Neuronal circuitry throughout the brain is designed to prevent constant electrical discharge. Activity in one neuron often projects to cells that either inhibit activity in adjacent neurons (surround inhibition) or inhibit activity of the same neuron (feedback inhibition). Many EEG rhythms are believed to be generated with the help of feedback inhibition. Afferent axons activate cortical neurons, which promotes efferent outflow. The cortical efferents project to the generator of afferent activity. By feedback inhibition this efferent activity inhibits cortical afferent activity and thereby reduces cortical activation. When feedback inhibition is lost, afferents again activate the cortex, completing the cycle. The afferent generator for the occipital alpha rhythm is thought to be the thalamus. Afferent generators for other rhythms may be the thalamus, other subcortical nuclei, and associative regions of the cortex.

Rhythms of 10 Hz and slower are probably generated by moderate-intensity synchronous cortical input. Faster frequencies may be generated by less synchronous input. This occurs when the cortex is not entrained to the afferent impulses but is instead undergoing sustained depolarization. Direct recordings from the cortex show a negative direct current (DC) potential. Routine EEG recordings do not show the DC shift because the low-frequency filter blocks detection of DC potentials.

Scalp Potentials

Scalp electrodes are not able to detect all of the charge movement occurring on the cortical surface. One estimate suggests that 6 cm^2 of cortical surface area must be synchronously activated for a potential to be recorded at the scalp. Potentials are volume-conducted through the meninges, skull, and scalp before they are picked up by the surface electrodes.

Scalp potentials are determined by the vectors of cortical activity. If the superficial layers of the cortex have a positive field potential and the deeper layers have a negative field potential, then the vector is vertical, with the positive end pointing toward the scalp electrodes. The amplitude of the vector depends on the total area of activated cortex and the degree of synchrony between cortical neurons. Scalp electrodes are not able to record electrical activity in deep nuclei. Their effective recording depth is only a few millimeters.

Generation of Epileptiform Activity

Epileptiform activity is generated when depolarization of the cortex results in synchronous activation of many neurons. It is conceptually attractive to equate action potentials and EEG spikes, but action potentials occur normally. The abnormality in epileptiform activity is the degree of synchrony. The physiological basis for spikes will first be presented, followed by a discussion of the mechanisms for EEG synchrony.

Spikes and Sharp Waves

Epileptiform activity consists predominantly of spikes and sharp waves. Spikes have a duration of less than 70 ms while sharp waves have a duration of 70 to 200 ms. Scalp recordings occasionally show only rhythmic slow activity or background suppression during a seizure. In this circumstance, the spikes are probably too deep within the brain to be in recording range of surface electrodes.

Spike potentials are the summation of synchronous EPSPs and action potentials in the cortex. Most of the electrical activity is due to EPSPs, since charge flow with action potentials is small. Depolarization of the superficial layers is associated with influx of sodium ions into the cells. This produces a surface negative field potential. Depolarization of the superficial layers is electrotonically conducted into deeper layers, where it produces a positive field potential. The dipole produced in this manner is similar to that discussed previously for EEG rhythms.

Typically, the negative end of the dipole points toward the cortical surface. While there are extensive convolutions to the brain, the most superficial cortical tissue is oriented parallel to the skull and scalp. Therefore, spikes and sharp waves are predominantly negative on scalp electrodes.

The negative end of the dipole can be detected by several surface electrodes, although there is usually a region of maximum voltage. The distribution of the potential across the cortical surface is called a *field*. These relationships are presented in Figure 9.3.

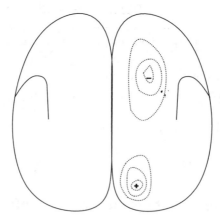

Figure 9.3 Cortical fields of a dipole. The negative (–) and positive (+) ends of a dipole are shown. This is the usual circumstance in which both ends can be seen on the surface. Usually, the positive end of the dipole is subcortical and cannot be recorded using surface electrodes. The dotted lines indicate zones of similar positivity or negativity, similar to altitude isobars on topographical maps of the earth.

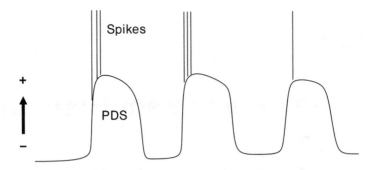

Figure 9.4   Paroxysmal depolarization shift. An electrode is in a pyramidal tract neuron. The slow waves are the PDS. The vertical lines represent action potentials superimposed on the PDS when the membrane potential reaches threshold.

Spikes and sharp waves are occasionally surface positive. Positive sharp waves are common in intraventricular hemorrhage of the newborn, and in two normal patterns: "14 and 6" Hz positive spikes and positive occipital sharp transients of sleep (POSTS).

Paroxysmal Depolarization Shifts

Paroxysmal depolarization shifts (PDS) are extracellular field potentials characterized by waves of depolarization followed by repolarization (Figure 9.4). High amplitude afferent input to the cortex produces depolarization of cortical neurons sufficient to trigger repetitive action potentials, which in turn contribute to the potential recorded at the surface. Repolarization, due to inactivation of interneurons, is followed by a brief period of hyperpolarization.

Cyclic depolarization and repolarization is believed to be the intracortical counterpart of the rhythmic spike activity seen in epilepsy. Rhythmicity is probably caused by the inability of cortical neurons to sustain prolonged high-frequency discharges. This is not caused by exhaustion but is a built-in mechanism of inactivation after sustained discharge.

10 ⬜⬜⬜
⬜⬜⬜
⬜⬜⬜

Technical Requirements for Electroencephalography

In 1986, the American Electroencephalographic Society published guidelines for performance of electroencephalograms (EEGs) and evoked potentials (EPs), which will be referred to here as the *Guidelines* (American Electroencephalographic Society 1986). This section summarizes the essentials of the technical requirements and offers suggestions for optimizing the acquisition of data.

Electroencephalography Equipment

Although at least eight channels of EEG are needed to sample activity from broad regions of the brain, sixteen channels are preferable and are now considered the real minimum for EEG. Sixteen channels allow the development of an accurate topographic map of EEG activity across both hemispheres but do not provide for the measurement of other physiological functions. A seventeenth channel is usually needed for the electrocardiogram (EKG) recording and additional channels are often useful to record other physiological functions, such as eye movements and respiration. Eye movement potentials are often recorded on EEG channels and can be misinterpreted as frontal slow wave activity. Respiratory movement produces periodic artifacts on the EEG channel. These physiological artifacts are best identified by simultaneously monitoring these functions.

The equipment available to record EEG activity has not changed substantially in recent years. The relatively expensive paperless EEGs not in general use, despite its advantages. Direct recording from individual electrodes provides the opportunity to inspect the same waveform in several different montages, since montages are created during playback. Further, paperless recordings are more environmentally sound and reduce storage needs.

In summary, if you are buying equipment for a diagnostic laboratory, sixteen channels are the minimum and twenty-one channels are desirable. Factors to consider in buying an EEG machine include:

1. *Price:* Cost considerations do not justify the purchase of an eight- or ten-channel machine. This is false economy. The difference in cost between an eight- and a sixteen-channel machine is more than offset by technician and physician time involved in obtaining an EEG of limited diagnostic utility.
2. *Portability:* The demand to transport hospital-based EEG machines to special care units is increasing. Such machines must be easy to move and constructed to withstand the movement.
3. *Technician familiarity:* It is preferable for all machines in one laboratory to be of the same brand, and even of the same series. Technicians alternating between brands are more likely to make mistakes and are less efficient.
4. *Service:* EEG machines frequently need service. Poor service support is an absolute contraindication to purchasing a machine. For many busy laboratories, service is a more important factor than performance specifications.

Specific Electroencephalographs

Most electroencephalographs are more than adequate for routine EEG. The author's laboratories have used Grass and Nihon-Kohden machines in a variety of models and configurations. In addition, other manufacturers make fine machines.

Grass

Grass electroencephalographs are sturdy and reliable. We use Grass machines mainly for portable studies. They are somewhat heavy, but little affected by the bumps and rattles of transport. Also, we have had better luck teaching nurses and residents how to use the Grass than other machines. The recordings are good; however, for uncertain reasons we find it easier to achieve low noise recordings with Nihon-Kohden.

Nihon-Kohden

Nihon-Kohden machines are well-built machines that we use predominantly for office and hospital laboratory studies. We have had some difficulty with pens coming out of alignment when the machines are moved, so we do not routinely use them for portable studies. Also, the amplifiers are below the paper deck, placing them at risk for the "Pepsi syndrome"—if drinks are placed on the paper, liquid can spill into the electronics. This is less likely in Grass machines, where the amplifiers are above and behind the paper platform.

Recommended Electrodes and Montages

Electrodes

The *Guidelines* recommends electrodes that do not attenuate frequencies between 0.5 and 70 Hz. Silver-silver chloride electrodes were among the first to be used because they produced little polarization. However, silver-silver chloride electrodes are expensive and have to be chlorided. Modern amplifiers have a very high input impedance and allow the use of other electrode materials. High impedance reduces the flow of current and reduces the opportunity for electrode polarization.

Commercial electrodes are preferable to homemade electrodes. Homemade electrodes have a greater potential for variable impedances and surface areas that may increase noise and adversely influence the recorded signal.

Surface Electrodes

Surface electrodes are used routinely for almost all EEG studies. Surface electrodes are silver or gold disks that are fixed to the skin with electrode gel, a viscous solution containing ions that can carry charge. The gel acts as a malleable extension of the electrode. Details of the function of electrodes are presented in part I on basic electronics and are in the article by Misulis (1989).

Application of surface electrodes using electrode gel involves the following steps:

1. Locate positions for electrodes using the "10-20 Electrode Placement System" (explained later in this chapter).
2. Separate strands of hair over the electrode positions using the wood end of a cotton-tipped applicator.
3. Clean dead skin and dirt from the region with Omni-prep® (D. O. Weaver Co., Denver, CO) using the cotton-tip applicator.
4. Scoop some gel into the electrode.
5. Place the electrode in position over the skin.
6. Put a 2" × 2" gauze pad over the electrode and push it firmly onto the head.

This action provides a good seal, preventing the electrode from falling off in all but the most vigorous head movements.

Application of electrodes with collodion involves the following steps:

1. Prepare the head as mentioned for electrode gel.

2. Place the electrode on the scalp.
3. Place a piece of gauze soaked with collodion over the electrode.
4. Use compressed air to dry the collodion.
5. Insert a blunt-tipped needle into the cup and score the skin, to lower electrode impedance.
6. Inject electrolyte into the cup of the electrode using the blunt-tipped needle.

Each method has its advantages. Collodion provides a much more secure attachment and is more suitable for long-term recordings. Electrode gel is easier to apply and remove, and is suitable for most routine office and hospital recordings.

Needle Electrodes

Needle electrodes offer no advantages over conventional surface electrodes and should not be used for routine studies. The risk of infection to the patient and technician is unacceptably high.

Sphenoidal Electrodes

Sphenoidal electrodes are used to evaluate patients with suspected temporal lobe seizures. They are inserted adjacent to the zygoma until they reach the base of the skull. Sphenoidal electrodes should only be used by physicians who are trained in their insertion and experienced in interpretation of the recorded potentials.

Subdural Strip Electrodes

Subdural strip electrodes are used to evaluate patients for epilepsy surgery. A burr hole or small craniotomy is performed and the electrode strips placed overlying the cortex, usually in the area immediately overlying the suspected seizure focus. The purpose is to map the anatomical extent of the focus.

Subdural strip electrodes should only be used by investigators experienced in their placement and recording interpretation and then only for preoperative evaluation before surgery for epilepsy.

Depth Electrodes

Depth electrodes are used to localize a seizure focus in patients being evaluated for surgery. Each electrode probe inserted into the brain is actually an array of small electrodes from which individual recordings are made. The position of the electrode is determined by skull radiographs and by correlation with computerized tomography. Depth electrodes should only be used by physicians trained in their insertion and recording interpretation.

Electrode Position

Electrodes should be placed according to the "10-20 Electrode Placement System," as recommended by the International Federation of Societies for EEG and Clinical Neurophysiology. This system uses twenty-one electrodes placed at positions that are measured at 10% and 20% of head circumference (Figure 10.1). The head is measured in the following manner:

1. Measure the distance from nasion to inion across the vertex. Mark a line at 50% of this distance.
2. Measure the distance between the preauricular points, just in front of the ear. Mark a line at 50% of this distance. The intersection of this line with that of Step 1 is Cz.
3. Lay the measuring tape from nasion to inion through Cz. Mark 10% of this distance above the nasion for Fpz and above the inion for Oz. Fz is 20% of this distance above Fpz. Pz is 20% of this distance above Oz.
4. Lay the tape between the preauricular points through Cz. T3 is 10% of this distance above the left preauricular point, and T4 is 10% above the right. C3 is 20% of this distance above T3, and C4 is 20% of this distance above T4.

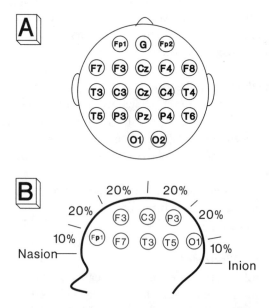

Figure 10.1   10-20 Electrode Placement System. *(A)* Top view. This diagram is similar to that seen on EEG paper. Nose is at the top, with the lateral protrusions representing ears. Circles with letters indicate electrodes and are meant more to be indicators of relative positions than exact positions. *(B)* Side view. Lines for measurement are shown. See text for details.

5. Lay the tape from Fpz to Oz through C3. F3 is 25% of this distance posterior to Fpz. P3 is 25% of this distance anterior to Oz. Move the tape to the same position on the right side, through C4, to mark F4 and P4.
6. Lay the tape from Fpz to Oz through T3. F7 is 25% of this distance posterior to Fpz. T5 is 25% of this distance anterior to Oz. Move the tape to the right side and measure in the same manner for F8 and T6.
7. Lay the tape from F7 to F8 through Fz, F3, and F4 to ensure that the distance between electrodes is equal. Then lay the tape from T5 to T6 through Pz, P3, and P4 in the same manner.

The terminology of electrode position is based on a key letter that indicates the brain region, and a number that specifies the exact position. The key letters are: *F* for frontal, *Fp* for fronto-polar, *C* for central, *T* for temporal, *P* for parietal, *O* for occipital, and *A* for auricular (ear). The numbers indicate the electrodes within the specified region. Odd numbers are on the left and even numbers are on the right. In general, lower numbers are anterior and higher numbers are posterior. Midline electrodes are indicated by *z* instead of by a number.

Abbreviations for special electrodes, such as *Sp* for sphenoidal and *Naso* for nasopharyngeal, are less standardized and may vary between laboratories. Subdural strip and depth electrodes often use both numbers and letters; the letter generally indicates the array and the numbers indicate which electrode in the array.

Montages

The sequence of electrodes being recorded at one time is called a *montage*. All montages fall into one of two categories: bipolar or referential (see Figure 10.2). *Referential* means that the reference for each electrode is in common with other electrodes; for example, each electrode may be referenced to the ipsilateral ear. An average reference means that each electrode is compared to the average potential of every electrode. *Bipolar* means that the reference for one channel is the active for the next; for example, in the longitudinal bipolar montage, channel 1 is Fp1-F3. This means that Fp1 is the active electrode and F3 is the reference. Channel 2 is F3-C3, so that F_3 is now the active electrode and C3 is the reference.

For all channels, negativity in the active input produces an upward deflection of the pen on the paper. Negativity at the reference produces downward deflection. Details of localization are discussed in chapter 11, "Electroencephalography Basics."

The *Guidelines* recommends the following principles in designing montages:

1. Record at least eight channels.
2. Use the full twenty-one electrode placement of the 10–20 system.

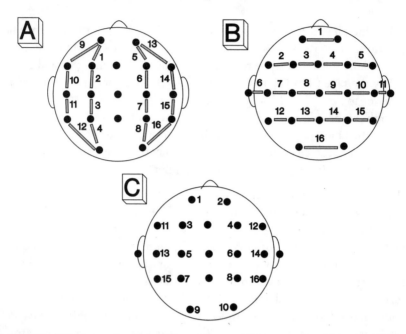

Figure 10.2 Bipolar and referential montages. *(A)* Longitudinal bipolar (LB) montage. *(B)* Transverse bipolar (TB) montage. *(C)* Referential montage. Only the active input (G_1) is shown. The electrodes could be referenced to the ear or to an average. For all of these, the number near the electrode position indicates channel number. The line represents the comparison of two adjacent electrodes in bipolar montages. G_1 is anterior and/or left of G_2.

3. Every routine recording session should include at least one montage from each of the following groups: referential (R), longitudinal bipolar (LB), and transverse bipolar (TB).
4. Label each montage on the recording.
5. Use simple montages that allow easy visualization of the spatial orientation of waveforms, that is, bipolar montages should be in straight lines with equal interelectrode distances.
6. List the anterior and left-sided channels before posterior and right-sided channels.
7. Use at least some montages that are commonly used in other laboratories.
8. Negativity in the active electrode of each channel produces an upward deflection of the pen.

The recommended sixteen-channel montages for routine use in adults are displayed in Table 10.1. Additional channels, when available, are used for monitoring other biological functions such as EKG, eye movements, respirations, and EMG, or for recording from the midline.

Table 10.1 Recommended Montages for Routine Electroencephalogram in Adults

Channel No.	LB	TB	Ave	Ref
1	Fp1-F3	Fp1-Fp2	Fp1-Ave	Fp1-A1
2	F3-C3	F7-F3	Fp2-Ave	Fp2-A2
3	C3-P3	F3-Fz	F3-Ave	F3-A1
4	P3-O1	Fz-F4	F4-Ave	F4-A2
5	Fp2-F4	F4-F8	C3-Ave	C3-A1
6	F4-C4	A1-T3	C4-Ave	C4-A2
7	C4-P4	T3-C3	P3-Ave	P3-A1
8	P4-O2	C3-Cz	P4-Ave	P4-A2
9	Fp1-F7	Cz-C4	O1-Ave	O1-A1
10	F7-T3	C4-T4	O2-Ave	O2-A2
11	T3-T5	T4-A2	F7-Ave	F7-A1
12	T5-O1	T5-P3	F8-Ave	F8-A2
13	Fp2-F8	P3-Pz	T3-Ave	T3-A1
14	F8-T4	Pz-P4	T4-Ave	T4-A2
15	T4-T6	P4-T6	T5-Ave	T5-A1
16	T6-O2	O1-O2	T6-Ave	T6-A2

LB = Longitudinal bipolar; TB = Transverse bipolar; Ave = Average reference; Ref = Ear reference.

Note: These montages are for a sixteen-channel machine. If a seventeenth channel is available, it is usually used for EKG. If twenty-one channels are available, additional channels are particularly useful for the LB montage. Extra channels may be Fz-Cz, Cz-Pz, and eye leads.

Source: American Electroencephalographic Society 1986.

Montages selected for children are age-dependent. The entire 10–20 electrode placement can be used in term newborns, but is not routinely needed. Monitoring noncerebral functions such as EKG and respiration are essential in all newborns and special montages must be used when only sixteen channels are available. Specific recommendations for neonatal EEG are presented in chapter 17, "Neonatal Electroencephalography."

Routine Electroencephalography

All recordings should be clearly labeled with the patient's name, age, recording date, identification number, and name of the technologist performing the recording. This should be done before the record leaves the recording room, to avoid mixing up of records from different patients. A face sheet accompanying the record should include reason for the study, time of last seizure (if applicable), technical summary, and annotation of regions to which the technician wants to call particular attention. Current medications should also be listed.

Calibration

Two phases of calibration are performed before starting the study. The first is square wave calibration and the second is biological calibration (Biocal).

Square-Wave Calibration
A square-wave pulse is delivered to the inputs of each amplifier. The pulse is 50 µV amplitude, alternating on and off at one-second intervals. The waveform is modified by the preset filters and recorded on paper. Sample square-wave calibration recordings are shown in Figure 10.3.

The low-frequency filter (LFF) transforms the plateau of the square wave into an exponential decay. The high-frequency filter (HFF) slightly rounds off the peak of the calibration pulse signal. For educational purposes, I recommend trying several different high- and low-frequency filter settings during the calibration test, in order to see the effect of filter changes on the record. It is also instructive to change filter settings during the recording of EEG activity, at a time that will not interfere with clinical interpretation.

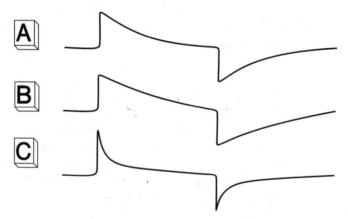

Figure 10.3 Square-wave calibration signals. A 50 µV square wave was delivered and the response recorded. *(A)* Normal response. *(B)* Increased time constant of the low-frequency filter. The potential decays slower than normal. *(C)* Decreased time constant of the low-frequency filter. The potential decays faster than normal.

The time constant (TC) of the LFF can be measured from the square-wave calibration page. As we said in part I, TC is equal to the time it takes for a potential to fall to 1/e of the original value, where e is the base of natural logarithms (approximately 2.7). Therefore, TC will be the time to decay to 37% of peak value, approximately ⅓ of the peak voltage.

It is difficult to estimate the setting of the HFF from the square-wave calibration; however, electroencephalographers should have an idea of what the peak should look like. If the HFF is set too low, there will be a slow roll-off on the peak of the calibration pulse. If the HFF is set too high, the wave will appear too peaked, and may even show overshoot, as if there is too little pen damping.

Biological Calibration

Biocal assesses the response of the amplifiers, filters, and the recording apparatus to a complex biological signal. Electrodes Fp1 and O2 are connected to all amplifier inputs. The recordings from all channels should be identical (Figure 10.4).

Pen Pressure and Damping

Mechanical writing instruments have two inherent limitations: inertia and friction. Even when the filters are set properly, the frequency response may be inaccurate because of these mechanical factors. The physical mass of the pen produces inertia that slows its response time to sudden changes in signal voltage. Inertia is partially compensated for by control mechanisms in the pen drive mechanism. Friction is also compensated by EEG-machine electronics, but excessive pressure of the pen on the paper results in a sluggish re-

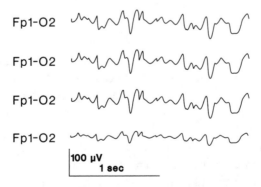

Figure 10.4 Bio-Calibration signals. Four channels are shown, all of which have the same input, that is, Fp1-O2. The trace from every channel should be identical; however, the last channel has a smaller amplitude response. This indicates unequal amplification and would be corrected before performing the study.

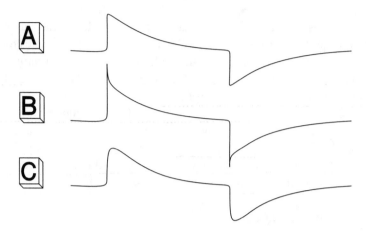

Figure 10.5 Pen damping. *(A)* Normal damping. *(B)* Under-little damping. Note the overshoot in the deflection on the rising phase of the calibration pulse. *(C)* Overdamping. Note the blunted response at the rising phase of the calibration pulse.

sponse. This is the main reason why electroencephalographers and technicians need a visual memory of what a calibration pulse looks like with proper filter settings.

The same inertia that inhibits pen movement also promotes excessive pen movement (overshoot). Overshoot is minimized by the pen control mechanism, termed *damping*. When damping is not sufficient, normal waveforms may look like spike discharges (Figure 10.5). These effects are minimized with proper setting of pen pressure and damping. The manuals provided with the EEG machines give instructions on setting the damping and pen pressure.

Sensitivity

The sensitivity is initially set at 7 µV/mm and subsequently adjusted depending on the amplitude of the EEG activity. Movement artifact and other noncerebral transients may exceed maximal pen excursion, but electrocerebral activity may not. Important waveforms may be missed when sensitivity is set too low.

In children, sensitivity is often reduced to 10 to 15 µV/mm because EEG amplitude is high in both the awake and sleep states. The elderly often have low-voltage EEG activity and increased sensitivity is required.

Studies performed for the determination of cerebral death are started at 7 µV/mm but the sensitivity is always increased to 2 µV/mm (see chapter 16, "Cerebral Death Studies").

Filters

The standard filter settings for routine EEG are LFF = 1 Hz and HFF = 70 Hz. These settings indicate the frequencies at which there is a 3-dB decrement. The LFF setting of 1 Hz corresponds to a time constant of 0.16 sec. See part I for a detailed discussion of filters.

If the LFF is set higher than 1 Hz, there will be attenuation and distortion of some slow waves. Slow waves have an increased number of phases and are composed of faster frequencies. Technicians should be discouraged from turning up the LFF, especially when there is an abundance of slow activity. If the HFF is set too low, then faster activity is blunted, and spikes and sharp waves may be impossible to identify.

The 60-Hz filter should not be needed in properly designed laboratories. Two important design features are careful selection of equipment location and adequate grounding. Shielding of the room is desirable but usually not essential; it cannot completely abolish artifact induced by a strong electromagnetic field. Studies in a special care unit usually require use of the 60-Hz filter. Sources of artifact include ventilators, intravenous infusion pumps, air beds, heating/cooling blankets, and monitoring equipment.

Duration of Recording

A routine EEG should include at least twenty minutes of relatively artifact-free record. Longer duration recordings are often helpful in neonates, so that transitions between states can be identified. The *Guidelines* recommends thirty minutes of recording for cerebral death studies.

Activation Methods

The performance and interpretation of records obtained with activation methods are discussed in detail in chapter 13, "Activation Methods." Hyperventilation, photic stimulation, and sleep may activate epileptiform activity. After an initial period of recording in the relaxed, wakeful state, the patient is asked to hyperventilate for three minutes. If absence seizures are suspected, the patient is asked to hyperventilate for five minutes. Hyperventilation is not performed in elderly individuals or in patients with advanced atherosclerotic disease, because of concern over vasoconstriction with resultant cardiac or cerebral hypoperfusion.

Photic stimulation is performed on older children and adults of all ages. Photic stimulation of sleeping infants is probably of no clinical value.

Sleep is not considered by some to be a true activation method, because it is a transition between natural states. However, sleep does help to promote epileptiform activity, and in routine EEG sleep frequently has to be induced by sedatives or sleep deprivation. In this sense, sleep is an activation method. Sleep recordings are routinely indicated in all patients being evaluated for seizures but are not helpful in patients being evaluated for encephalopathy. The mechanism of sleep is not important. There is no convincing evidence that natural sleep, sedated sleep, and sleep deprivation differ in their ability to promote epileptiform activity.

Telephone Transmission Electroencephalography

Telephone transmission of EEG is useful and accurate with certain caveats. The interpreter must be aware of several sources of artifact from public telephone lines and the equipment required to transform the data into a form for transmission.

The EEG signal is carried from one institution to another across a single telephone line. Therefore, the signal is multiplexed. *Multiplexing* means that the line carries brief samples of each channel in turn. A voltage measurement of channel 1 is followed by channel 2 then 3, and so on. After the last channel, an additional channel is often transmitted for error checking and comment information. Then, voltage for channel 1 is transmitted and the cycle begins again. At the receiving end, the multiplexed signal is reconstructed into separate channels and displayed on EEG paper.

The *Guidelines* recommends that telephone transmission EEGs be performed in accordance with the guidelines for routine EEGs, and in addition make the following recommendations:

1. Manufacturers of telephone transmission EEG equipment must provide specifications on frequency response, noise, and crosstalk. The equipment should be checked periodically to ensure that these specifications are continually met.
2. The equipment should indicate if there is difficulty with transmission at either station or in the telephone transmission itself.
3. Integrity of transmission should be checked before and after each recording.
4. The record should be labeled as already described. In addition, the record should indicate that it is a telephone transmission recording.
5. A paper recording should be made at both the transmitting and receiving stations, for accurate relay of information on physiological state, activity, and artifacts.
6. The EEG from both transmitting and receiving stations should be stored for future comparison.

7. The technicians at the transmitting and receiving stations should be well trained not only in routine EEG, but also in the techniques and problems associated with telephone transmission EEGs.
8. Telephone transmission EEG cannot be used as a confirmatory test for determination of brain death.

Technicians at outside facilities are seldom as well trained and supervised as technicians in the home EEG laboratory. Therefore, there is greater opportunity for technical error. Many outside facilities use electrode caps. These caps fit snugly on the head. There are several problems with electrode caps: (1) impedances are usually higher than with normally applied electrodes; (2) the cap may not be positioned perfectly on the head; and (3) the relative positions of the electrodes differ between patients because of head size.

The Electroencephalography Laboratory

EEGs can be performed in virtually any patient care area of a hospital, but routine studies are best performed in a central EEG laboratory. Because sleep is a requisite part of many studies, the EEG laboratory should be located in a quiet area. Many experts recommend locating the EEG machine in a room adjacent to the patient room, so that technician and equipment noise do not interfere with performance of the study. In practice, this isolation is not usually needed and does not warrant the added construction costs.

All laboratory outlets should accept a three-prong plug and be properly grounded. Improper grounding is the most common cause of shock hazard. All patients equipment must be grounded to a common point that is functioning well (see chapter 8 on electrical safety).

Electrical shielding is usually not necessary and should not be installed routinely. Excessive interference is more likely to result from improper grounding or electrode problems than from the environment. With adequate grounding and the use of bipolar montages, good recordings can be made in most facilities.

Electroencephalography Reports and Recordkeeping

The EEG Report

The EEG report must be complete, clear, and concise (Figure 10.6). It should be no longer than one page, not including representative samples of the record. Every record must have the following information: patient name, hospital or laboratory unit number, EEG record number, date of study, age, sex, reason for study, current medications, time of last seizure (if

---

St. Nowhere's Hospital Neurophysiology Laboratory

```
Name:        John Doe       Date:   1/2/92
Hospital #:  1234567        Age:    30              Sex:  M
Physician:   A. Brown
```

Study: Electroencephalogram - wake and sleep

Clinical: Tonic-clonic seizures. Last 12/30/91.

Medications: Dilantin 300 mg qhs. Last dose 11pm 1/1/92.

Description:
     The recording begins with the patient in the waking state
and is characterized by a posterior dominant rhythm of 10 Hz that
attenuates to eye opening. There is an anterior-posterior
gradient with faster frequencies from the frontal regions.
     The patient was sedated with 1 gm of chloral hydrate and
stage 2 sleep was obtained. The sleeping state was characterized
by well-formed vertex waves and sleep spindles.
     No focal or epileptiform abnormalities were seen.

Interpretation:
     Normal wake and sleep EEG.

                                              Joe Smith, M.D.

Figure 10.6 Sample EEG report.

applicable), description of the record, interpretation, and name of the electro-encephalographer.

Description of the Record

The description is the body of the report. This section is not read by many referring physicians but will be used by neurologists who may want the evidence supporting the final impression. It will also be used for comparison with future studies. The essential elements of the description include state of the patient including state transitions during the study, description of the background and reactivity, and response to activation methods.

A description of a normal record might read as follows:

EEG #1: The recording began with the patient in the awake state, and was characterized by a posterior dominant rhythm of 10 Hz, which reacted to eye opening. Hyperventilation for 3 min produced symmetric slowing. Photic stimulation produced a driving response at flash frequencies of 9–18/sec. The patient was sedated with 1 gm of chloral hydrate and stage 2 sleep was obtained. The sleeping state was characterized by symmetric sleep spindles, vertex waves, and slow activity in the theta and delta range.

A description of an abnormal record might read as follows:

EEG #2: The recording began with the patient in the awake state and was characterized by a posterior dominant rhythm of 9 Hz which reacted to eye opening. Posterior slow waves of youth are superimposed on the record. During the waking state, generalized 3/sec spike wave complexes were seen with maxima in the frontal regions. Duration of the discharges was 2 to 7 seconds. Hyperventilation augmented the spike wave complexes. Photic stimulation produced a driving response at flash frequencies of 7–15/sec. The patient was sedated with 2 gm of chloral hydrate and became drowsy, but stage 2 sleep was not obtained.

The description is the location for any abnormalities or irregularities in the record. For example, a single spike may be seen which does not recur during the record. A conservative reader will hesitate to interpret a record as abnormal on the basis of a single spike. Therefore, the description may include the following passage:

EEG #3: . . . During the waking state, a single spike was observed with maximal negativity at C3. The spike did not recur during the record . . .

The final impression of this recording would be normal. If a future EEG showed more obvious epileptiform activity, the interpreter could look back at this report and conclude that the spike was consistent with the patient's known seizure disorder.

Interpretation

For the referring physician, the interpretation is the most important part of the report. First, state whether the record is normal or abnormal, then summarize the abnormalities, and conclude with the clinical implications of the abnormalities. Interpretations for the EEGs described above are as follows:

EEG #1: Normal awake and sleep EEG.

EEG #2: Abnormal EEG because of generalized 3/sec spike wave complexes. This is consistent with a seizure disorder of the generalized type.

Ordinarily, the EEG interpretation should provide a definitive diagnosis that requires no further interpretation by the clinician. However, sometimes the EEG interpretation can be further refined by clinical data. Usually, the clinical neurophysiologist does not know the patient but is in the best position to interpret the clinical significance of the EEG. Some examples are:

Finding #1: Spike focus in a patient with partial complex seizures.

Impression #1: "This is an abnormal study because of a spike focus in the right anterior temporal region. This is consistent with a partial seizure disorder."

Finding #2: Sharp wave focus in a patient with a behavioral disorder.

Impression #2: "This is an abnormal study because of a sharp wave focus in the left posterior temporal region. While this could be consistent with a seizure disorder, patients without clinical seizures may manifest this pattern."

Electroencephalography Recordkeeping

The *Guidelines* gives no recommendations regarding keeping EEG records and reports. It is not practical to keep permanently the entirety of every EEG record. Options to archive records include microfilming the entire record or saving representative paper sheets. Microfilm is preferable, because selected samples may not accurately reflect the entire record. Private services are available nationwide to microfilm EEG records. For a nominal fee, they arrange for pickup of the records and return a cataloged film. The cost and efficiency of these services makes them preferable to owning equipment for all but the largest laboratories.

State-of-the-art digital EEG machines record signals on magnetic or optical disk, or tape. The amount of digitized information is massive, considering the sampling speed required for twenty-one channels of at least a twenty-minute recording. As a result, the cost of digital recording is usually greater than that of microfilm. This cost is quickly declining with advances in technology. Digital EEG recording will probably be a future standard.

The EEG report should be kept indefinitely. Hospital-based laboratories must follow institutional and state requirements for recordkeeping.

11 ⬜⬜⬜
⬜⬜⬜
⬜⬜⬜

Electroencephalography Basics

Clinical Indications for Electroencephalography

The situations in which electroencephalographic (EEG) studies are most useful are seizures, encephalopathy, encephalitis, and brain death. Modern imaging studies have reduced the usefulness of EEG in the evaluation of headache and focal neurologic disturbances.

Electroencephalographic Rhythms

Electroencephalographic rhythms are classified into four frequency bands. No individual frequency band is normal or abnormal by definition. All are interpreted as normal or abnormal depending on the age and state of the patient.

Beta	> 13 Hz
Alpha	8–13 Hz
Theta	4–7 Hz
Delta	< 4 Hz

Alpha

The alpha rhythm is usually seen in normal, relaxed individuals who are awake with their eyes closed. It is approximately 10 Hz in adults with the maximum voltage recorded from the occipital electrodes, O1 and O2. The term *alpha rhythm* was once used to describe any posterior dominant waking rhythm, but this convention is no longer used.

In children, the dominant occipital rhythm is slower in frequency and may not attain 8.5 Hz until 12 years of age. Slower frequencies in a 12-year-old that are bilateral suggest an encephalopathy or, if unilateral, suggest a focal lesion.

The alpha rhythm is suppressed when the eyes are opened and promptly returns when the eyes are closed. This "reactivity" of the alpha rhythm should be tested routinely. The alpha rhythm is suppressed if the individual is tense during the recording and should not be interpreted as abnormal. Other EEG criteria that suggest a tense state are muscle artifact in frontal and temporal leads and frequent irregular eye-blink potentials.

The amplitude of the posterior alpha rhythm is 15 to 50 µV in young adults. In older individuals, the amplitude is often low, but the frequency is the same. Slowing of the posterior rhythm is not a normal part of aging. The frequency of the posterior rhythm in elderly individuals who are intellectually intact is the same as in middle-aged adults. Amplitude asymmetries of the posterior alpha rhythm are relatively common in normal people. The amplitude is usually higher from the nondominant hemisphere but should not exceed 50%. A prominent alpha rhythm may be recorded during general anesthesia and coma. The appearance of generalized alpha during coma (alpha coma) is usually associated with asphyxial encephalopathies and suggests a poor prognosis. Alpha activity during coma and anesthesia is more generalized than during the normal resting state and has an anterior predominance. The rhythm is monotonous and lacks the usual modulation of frequency and amplitude.

Beta

Electroencephalographic activity with frequencies faster than 13 Hz occurs in all individuals but is usually of low amplitude and often overlooked in favor of slower frequencies during wakefulness and sleep. Beta activity is normally distributed maximally over the frontal and central regions. A low-amplitude (25 µV) high-frequency (25 Hz) beta is especially prominent during normal sleep in infants and children, and is enhanced by several sedatives, especially barbiturates and benzodiazepines. In some sedated children, beta activity may be sufficiently prominent to obscure the record.

People with hyperthyroidism may accelerate their posterior rhythm from 10 to 14 Hz or faster. This is technically in the beta range, but the rhythm continues to react like an occipital, awake, resting rhythm and should be considered no different than an alpha rhythm.

Alterations in the frequency, amplitude, or abundance of beta activity should be commented upon in the description of the record but interpreted with caution. Marked asymmetry in beta activity suggests the possibility of a structural abnormality on the side lacking beta. Focal, high-amplitude beta activity can be recorded over a skull defect, such as burr holes and fracture sites (breach rhythm).

Theta

Electroencephalographic activity with a frequency between 4 and 8 Hz is seen in normal drowsiness and sleep, and during wakefulness in young children. Theta is also present in normal waking adults, but the content is small and the amplitude is low. The detection of this theta usually requires high-sensitivity recordings or digital-frequency analysis.

Posterior slow waves of youth may be in the theta or delta range. Theta activity in the temporal region in older individuals has been ascribed to vascular disease. While the significance of temporal theta is controversial, I suspect that it is not part of normal aging. I suggest commenting on the presence of temporal theta in the body of the report and interpreting it as a mild abnormality.

Delta

Delta activity is not normally recorded in the awake adult but is a prominent feature of sleep and becomes increasingly abundant during the progress from stage 2 to stage 4 sleep (see section on sleeping rhythms in chapter 12, "Normal Electroencephalography Patterns").

Focal polymorphic delta activity (PDA) may be recorded over localized regions of cerebral damage. Intermittent rhythmic delta activity is recorded when there is dysfunction of the relays between the deep gray matter and cortex. This activity has a frontal predominance in adults and is called frontal intermittent rhythmic delta activity (FIRDA), while in children the activity has an occipital predominance and is called occipital intermittent rhythmic delta activity (OIRDA) or posterior intermittent rhythmic delta activity (PIRDA).

Spikes and Sharp Waves

The mechanisms of generation of spikes and sharp waves were discussed in chapter 9. Spikes are usually surface negative. The positive end of the dipole is occasionally detected on the cortical surface distant from the region of greatest negativity.

Spikes and sharp waves usually indicate epileptiform activity; however, sharp waves are normal in certain situations, such as in newborns. Spikes and sharp waves are also seen overlying structural lesions, even in the absence of seizures. Interpretation of spikes and sharp waves is discussed in detail in chapter 14, "Spikes and Sharp Waves."

Slow Waves

Slowing can take two forms: (1) slow background rhythms; and (2) slow waves superimposed on the background. A posterior dominant rhythm of 7 Hz is abnormally slow and is consistent with an encephalopathy.

In contrast, focal slow waves in the theta and delta range superimposed on an otherwise normal background suggest a structural lesion. Interpretation of slow waves is discussed in detail in chapter 15, "Slow Activity."

Localization

Interpretation of the EEG depends on accurate localization of recorded electrical activity. Every potential has a field, although the extent of the field may not be within range or resolution limits of the electrodes. A field consists of a positive pole, a negative pole, and a distribution of the potential through the brain.

Localization is easiest with the average referential montage. In this montage, the reference for each channel is the average potential for all electrodes on the scalp. The left hemisphere portion of the most commonly used average referential montage is as follows:

Channel	Active	Reference
1	Fp1	Ref
3	F3	Ref
5	C3	Ref
7	P3	Ref
9	O1	Ref

By convention, negativity at the active electrode gives an upward deflection on routine EEG. For our hypothetical spike, maximal negativity is in channel 5, with lesser negativity in channels 3 and 7. Channels 1, 9, and all others not listed do not show the spike. Therefore, the spike focus is localized at C3.

On first inspection, bipolar montages make visual analysis more complex, but they facilitate precise spatial localization. The left parasaggital portion of the longitudinal bipolar (LB) montage is as follows:

Channel	Active	Reference
1	Fp1	F3
2	F3	C3
3	C3	P3
4	P3	O1

For the same spike as described for the average referential montage, channel 2 shows a downward deflection because of negativity at C3, the reference electrode. Channel 3 shows an upward deflection because C3 is the active electrode. The smaller spike at Channel 1 also points down, because of a lesser negativity at F3. Likewise, the small spike at channel 4 is upward because of negativity at P3. The appearance of this recording is that spikes point toward each other. The electrode where the direction of deflection changes is the most negative location of the spike. Bipolar montages can also allow for location of spikes even between electrode positions. Using the same LB montage, if a spike focus is between F3 and C3, the spike will point downward in channel 1 and upward in channel 3. Since the negativity is approximately equal in F3 and C3, there will be virtually no deflection.

Slow waves can be localized by polarity. However, slow waves are usually not as stereotyped as spikes. Therefore, localization depends more on absolute amplitude than polarity. The exception to this rule is differentiation of eye movement artifact from slow activity in the frontal lobes, discussed in detail in chapter 12.

12 Normal Electroencephalography Patterns

Specific electroencephalographic (EEG) waveforms are rarely normal or abnormal, with the exception of certain epileptiform discharges, but must be interpreted within the context of the patient's age and awake-sleep state. Delta activity is normal in sleep stages 3 and 4 and abnormal in coma. For the experienced electroencephalographer, the visual analysis is mainly automatic. The following starting points are recommended:

1. Note the patient's age, clinical state, medication list, and the reason for ordering the EEG.
2. Examine the composition of frequencies and their topographical organization, such as occipitally predominant alpha or frontal delta.
3. Examine the right-to-left symmetry of EEG patterns.
4. Examine systematic changes in EEG background during the recording.
5. Note abnormal waveforms such as spikes. Ask yourself if these could be normal waveforms.

EEG interpretation is subjective and difficult. Electroencephalographers need to have a conservative bias. Do not call an EEG abnormal if there is reasonable doubt. More harm is done by a false positive interpretation than by a false negative interpretation. Finally, do not hesitate to consult EEG texts when reviewing records that are difficult to interpret. For future reference, it may be helpful to cite supporting documentation in the impression.

Waking Rhythms

Normal Adult

Fast frequencies dominate the normal adult EEG in the awake, relaxed state when the eyes are closed. A posterior alpha rhythm is recorded

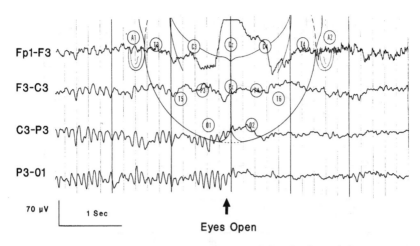

Figure 12.1 Normal EEG. Posterior dominant alpha rhythm of about 10 to 11 Hz. Only the first four channels of the longitudinal bipolar montage are shown.

with highest amplitude from the O1 and O2 electrodes (Figure 12.1). A central alpha rhythm may also be recorded, but it is usually of lower amplitude than that recorded from the occipital region. The background activity from the anterior region is composed predominantly of low-voltage fast activity with superimposed eye movement artifact. Rhythmic beta, especially when sedatives are used, may be recorded in the frontal and central regions. Drug-enhanced beta is more commonly seen following benzodiazepine and barbiturate sedation than following chloral hydrate. Theta and delta are not prominent in the normal awake adult EEG. However, digital frequency analysis shows a small amount of bihemispheric theta in most patients.

The occipital-predominant alpha is attenuated when the eyes are opened or when the patient is tense. An indication of patient tenseness is the recording of electromyographic (EMG) activity in the temporal regions from contraction of the masseter muscles. Electromyographic activity is faster in frequency and sharper in configuration than EEG activity.

Normal Child

Normal EEG patterns vary with age. The amplitude of potentials in children is generally greater than in adults. This applies not only to the posterior alpha, but especially to the frontal beta, which may be further enhanced by sedatives. Beta activity can be large enough to impair evaluation of other frequencies.

Theta activity is more prominent in children than in adults. Adolescents with 10-Hz posterior dominant rhythms will often have some bihemispheric

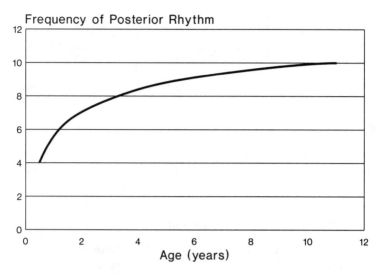

Figure 12.2   Maturation of the posterior dominant rhythm. Graph of frequency of the waking posterior dominant rhythm as a function of age.

theta that should be considered normal if the background is otherwise normal and the theta does not appear rhythmic.

Maturation of the Posterior Dominant Rhythm

The posterior dominant rhythm in the awake infant is approximately 4 Hz. The rhythm becomes faster with age, reaching the normal adult frequency of approximately 10 Hz by 10 years. This maturation is shown in Figure 12.2. The amplitude gradually increases, such that by age 10 the alpha is often more than 100 μV. In adults, the alpha amplitude gradually declines with increasing age.

Slow Waves of Youth

Slow waves of youth are in the delta range and are superimposed on the normal posterior dominant alpha rhythm. They are seen primarily in the waking state and occasionally in light drowsiness. Slow waves of youth may be differentiated from pathological slow waves by the otherwise normal background and their reactivity to eye opening. Slow waves of youth decrease with increasing age, and are not seen after the age of 30 years.

Sleeping Rhythms

Sleep promotes some epileptiform activity and is used as an activation method. However, the morphology of epileptiform discharges may

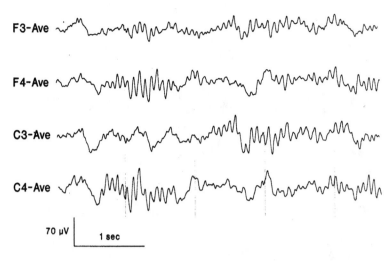

F3-Ave

F4-Ave

C3-Ave

C4-Ave

70 µV | 1 sec

Figure 12.3   Sleep spindles. The high frequency waveforms have a fronto-central predominance and are most prominent in stage 2 sleep.

look different in sleep when compared to the waking state. Sleep patterns differ in children and adults, and are discussed in the next section.

Normal Adult Sleep Patterns

The posterior dominant alpha rhythm of relaxed waking state attenuates with drowsiness. As the alpha disappears, theta activity appears from both hemispheres. This is commonly referred to as stage 1 sleep (see the section on sleep stages later in this chapter). Stage 2 sleep occurs when sleep spindles and vertex waves appear. These are the most common sleep stages seen in routine EEG. Deeper stages of sleep are rarely seen in routine daytime EEG. Below is a detailed description of sleep patterns and stages.

Vertex waves

Vertex waves are surface negative potentials with maximum amplitude at the midline (Cz). They are most common in stage 2 sleep and often appear at times of partial arousal.

Sleep spindles

Sleep spindles are rhythmic 11 to 14 Hz waves whose duration is typically 1 to 2 seconds (minimum is 0.5 sec) and whose amplitude is at least 25 µV (Figure 12.3). They are most prominent in the central regions during stage 2 sleep. Unlike vertex waves, the maximum amplitude of sleep

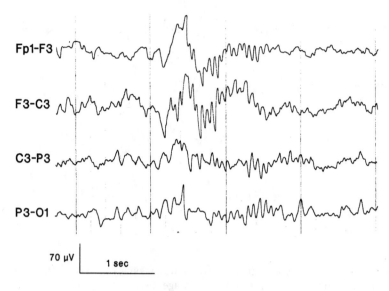

Figure 12.4   K complex. A K complex is the fusion of a vertex wave with a sleep spindle and is most characteristic of stage 2 sleep.

spindles is typically seen lateral to the midline (in the region of C3 and C4). Asymmetry in the abundance of sleep spindles is normal unless sleep spindles fail to appear from one hemisphere.

K Complexes

K complexes are formed by the fusion of sleep spindles and vertex waves (Figure 12.4). They are most commonly seen in stage 2 sleep and during partial arousal. They have no special significance beyond their individual elements.

Positive Occipital Sharp Transients of Sleep

Positive occipital sharp transients of sleep (POSTS) are surface positive potentials with maxima at O1 and O2. They may occur as single waves or in trains. They resemble lambda waves, except that they are present only in the sleeping state, whereas lambda waves are present only in the waking state with eyes open.

While POSTS may be related to a replaying of visual information, this hypothesis is not universally accepted. They are not seen in patients who are blind or severely visually impaired.

POSTS are not a constant feature of sleep and have no diagnostic significance, unless they are absent from only one side. This asymmetry is unlikely to be the only sign of focal abnormality in an EEG record.

Sleep Stages

Stage 1

Stage 1 is subdivided into stages 1A and 1B. Stage 1A is light drowsiness, characterized by attenuation of the alpha, slight slowing of the background, and spread of the alpha anteriorly. Stage 1B is characterized by less than 20% alpha with a predominance of slow activity in the theta range. Vertex waves may be seen in stage 1B, but are usually a sign of stage 2. Differentiation of 1A and 1B is not important for routine EEG.

Stage 2

Stage 2 sleep is characterized by sleep spindles, vertex waves, increased theta, and the appearance of delta. However, less than 20% of the record contains delta. Since some vertex waves can be seen in state 1B, the main differentiating feature is the appearance of sleep spindles.

Stage 3

Stage 3 sleep is characterized by increasing delta content and reduction in faster frequencies. Delta comprises 20% to 50% of the record.

Stage 4

Stage 4 sleep is characterized by a further increase in delta content, so that delta comprises more than 50% of the record. Vertex waves and sleep spindles are less prominent, and are often absent.

Rapid Eye Movement Sleep

Rapid eye movement (REM) sleep is characterized by a low-voltage background composed of predominantly fast frequencies. It can be difficult to distinguish REM sleep from light drowsiness. Rhythmic 6 to 8 Hz activity may appear in the frontal regions and vertex, which is called *sawtooth waves* because of its unusual morphology.

Typically, REM sleep follows after progression from sleep stages 1 through 4. Progression from drowsiness to REM sleep without passing through other stages (REM-onset sleep) occurs in patients with narcolepsy, after sleep deprivation, and after alcohol- or drug-induced REM-deprivation sleep.

The features of REM sleep that distinguish it from drowsiness are (1) rapid and chaotic eye movements (drowsiness is associated with slow roving eye movements), (2) hypotonia as measured by submental EMG, and (3) an irregular respiratory rate.

Sequence of Sleep Stages

The sequence of sleep stages for a normal adult is shown in part V, "Polysomnography." The cycle of sleep stages is repeated approximately three to four times per night, although there may not be progression to deeper stages with every cycle. Usually REM sleep occurs after at least one sleep cycle and increases in duration during subsequent cycles.

Respiratory pattern is usually regular in all sleep stages except REM. Submental EMG activity declines progressively as sleep becomes deeper until disappearing during REM sleep.

Changes in Sleep Stages with Age

Sleep patterns in children, after the neonatal period, are similar to those in adults. Neonatal sleep patterns are detailed in chapter 17 on neonatal EEG.

A child has normally identifiable sleep patterns by 1 year of age. Sleep spindles are present by 2 months and vertex waves by 5 months, although initial vertex waves have a blunted morphology. By 2 years of age, sleep spindles and vertex waves are abundant, sharp in configuration, and high in amplitude. Clusters of vertex waves may be mistaken for epileptiform activity. Later in childhood, vertex waves are less abundant but still high in amplitude. Sleep patterns continue to evolve throughout adult life.

Total hours of sleep declines and numbers of awakenings during sleep increase. Stages 3 and 4 become shorter, producing a reduced latency of REM sleep.

Normal Noncerebral Potentials

Noncerebral potentials can obscure normal cerebral potentials and can be mistaken for physiological potentials. Noncerebral potentials are of two types: (1) noncerebral potentials of physiologic origin, and (2) electrical artifact. The most prominent noncerebral physiologic potentials are from eye movement.

Eye Movement

Eye movement artifact is seen in anterior leads in virtually all records. The eye is polarized with the cornea being positive relative to the fundus. Therefore, when the eye rotates to look down, the leads over the frontal region are close to the negative end of the ocular dipole. This effect is most prominent for Fp1, Fp2, F3, and F4. The reverse is true with upward gaze; the frontal leads are close to the positive end of the dipole. With lateral gaze, the electrodes most affected are F7 and F8. For example, with left gaze, F7 becomes more positive while F8 becomes more negative.

Differentiating eye movement artifact from electrocerebral activity is usually not difficult. First, eye movements have a stereotypic pattern that looks different from most abnormal frontal slow activity, which is usually more polymorphic. The onset of slow waves caused by eye movement is rapid with a slower decay. Also, eye movement waveforms are typically superimposed on a normal low-voltage, high-frequency background. Abnormal frontal delta activity is usually associated with increased theta and reduced beta in the frontal regions. If identification is in doubt, eye leads should be placed to definitively distinguish between cerebral and eye activity.

Eye leads can be placed in several ways. The two most common methods are shown in Figure 12.5. We use method A. Electrodes are placed above and lateral to the right eye and below and lateral to the left eye. These electrodes are referenced to an average or ear electrode. With upward gaze, the positive end of the dipole rotates toward the right lead but away from the left. This causes pen deflections of opposite polarity in the recording. With left gaze, the positive cornea rotates toward the left lead but away from the right. Again, the pen deflections will be in opposite directions. These electrode derivations will detect slow activity in the frontal lobes, but this slow activity will not reverse between the two sides. Therefore, in these channels, slow activity that is opposite in polarity is of ocular origin, while slow activity that is of the same polarity on both sides is most likely of cerebral origin.

Method B of eye movement detection (Figure 12.5B) allows for precise determination of direction of gaze. Vertical gaze can be distinguished from horizontal gaze. This is seldom of interest on routine EEG testing.

Muscle Artifact

Electromyographic (EMG) activity is a frequent contaminant of EEG recordings. It is most prominent in the awake state, and is characterized by very fast, short duration spikes in the temporal and frontal regions (Figure 12.6). Amplitude is approximately 50 μV. Electromyographic activity is due to discharge of motor units in the temporalis and frontalis muscles. Distinction from spikes of cerebral origin is usually not difficult.

1. EMG activity is very fast. In fact, the predominant frequency is much faster than the high frequency filter setting of 70 Hz.
2. EMG activity is not followed by a slow wave.
3. EMG is most prominent in the waking, tense state, and disappears with relaxed wakefulness and sleep. In contrast, epileptiform activity is often best seen in drowsiness and sleep.

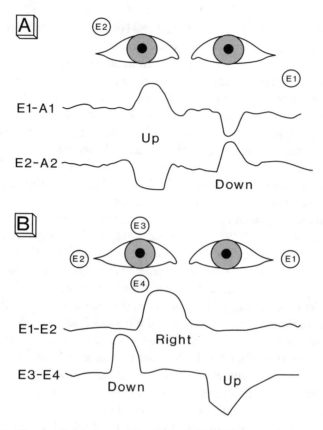

Figure 12.5 Eye lead placement. These leads help differentiate between eye movement and frontal slow activity. *(A)* Method used in our laboratory. *(B)* Alternative method.

4. EMG activity can often be attenuated by asking the patient to open his mouth. While the masseters and ptergoids do not contribute much to surface EMG activity, this relaxation allows for decreased activation of scalp muscles as well.

Electrocardiogram Artifact

Electrocardiogram (EKG) artifact is a frequent contaminant of EEG recordings and can be mistaken for epileptiform activity. It is most prominent with high sensitivities, ear reference montages, and in ICU recordings (Figure 12.7). Recording of EKG on a separate channel prevents confusion. If there is no "extra" channel, then the technician should sacrifice a channel during part of the recording, especially if sharp waveforms are seen.

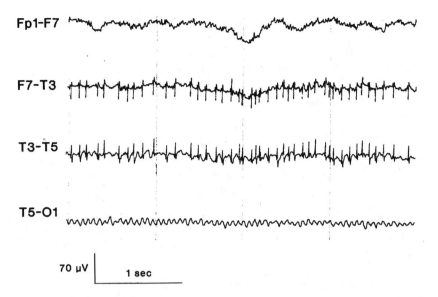

Figure 12.6 Muscle artifact. Fast activity in lateral leads is the surface recording of motor unit potentials.

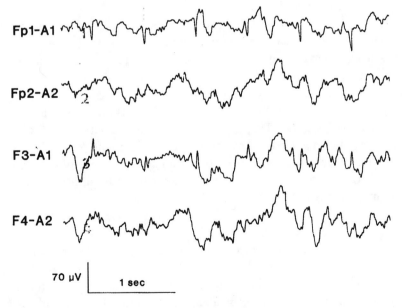

Figure 12.7 EKG artifact. The periodic sharp waves in channels 1 and 3 are due to contamination by EMG. This is most common in ear reference montages. A separate EMG channel was recorded but is not shown.

Glossokinetic Artifact

Glossokinetic artifact is due to tongue movement. The tongue is a dipole with the tip negative with respect to the base. Tongue movements in the waking state are seen in the EEG as delta activity, and can be mistaken for pathological frontal delta. Glossokinetic activity disappears with drowsiness and sleep.

Differentiation of glossokinetic artifact from electrocerebral slow activity can be difficult and may require technician observation. It is usually concurrent with muscle artifact of the temporalis and frontalis. If there is still any doubt, electrodes should be placed below the orbits. These electrodes are too distant to detect electrocerebral activity, but will pick up slow activity due to tongue or eye movement. The patient can be asked to say "la la la" so that the potential field and appearance of glossokinetic artifact can be identified.

Movement Artifact

Movement artifact was briefly discussed in part I, "Basic Electronics." There are two sources of movement artifact, electrode-gel interface and electrode leads.

Electrode-Gel Interface

A diffusion potential is established at the interface between the electrode and the gel, caused by movement of ions between the two substances. The concept is similar to the creation of a resting membrane potential in cell membranes. When there is movement of the electrodes, the junction is disturbed, and the junction potential discharges, injecting current through the electrode into the input amplifier. This is interpreted by the amplifier as a voltage pulse. This type of movement artifact looks like a brief spike followed by a gradual decay toward zero. During the pulse, the responsiveness of the amplifier may be reduced, since the amount of current flow from the artifact can be sufficient to overload the input amplifier. If there is no further movement, a new equilibrium is established.

Electrode Leads

The flow of electrons through electrical lines creates a weak magnetic field. Magnetic fields in turn can influence the flow of electrons through conductors, that is, they can induce current. This interaction between current and magnetic fields is termed *inductance* and is the physical basis for inductors, which were discussed in chapter 2. Inductance is also important for the generation of noise.

Electrode leads are unshielded and therefore susceptible to the effects of ambient magnetic fields. These magnetic fields are created by current in nearby power lines and equipment. Magnetic fields then induce current to flow through the electrode leads. The mechanism is termed *stray inductance*, because the inductance is not intentional within the machinery but rather unintentional. The induced current flows through the electrode leads just as signal current does. The amplifier cannot distinguish between signal and noise, so both are amplified. Since line power is 60 Hz, this creates 60-Hz interference.

The other major source of 60-Hz interference is *stray capacitance*. There is a small amount of capacitance between electrode leads and between leads and power lines. A charge can build up across this capacitance. The capacitance will change with electrode lead movement, thereby altering the built-up potential. Also, alternating current in power lines can create a small capacitative current in electrode leads, thereby creating 60-Hz interference.

The differential amplifier will reject much of the 60-Hz interference, however, the rejection is incomplete in the following conditions:

- If electrodes are affected unequally by stray inductance and stray capacitance (because of difference in lead position and proximity to electrical wires)
- If there are unequal electrode impedances
- If there is electrode movement.

When the electrodes are stable, stray inductance can cause 60-cycle interference that is rejected by the differential amplifiers. However, when there is electrode movement, the orientation of the electrode leads in space is altered. This produces a sudden change in induced current. The transient alteration in current is interpreted by the amplifier as a voltage shift.

Machine Artifact

This is discussed more under 60-Hz interference (part I, chapter 7). It is not "normal" but a frequent accompaniment to EEG recordings. The opportunity for machine artifact is greatest in the ICU. Figure 12.8 shows the artifact created by the motor of an air bed. The artifact disappears after the bed is unplugged.

Normal Variant Patterns

Mu Rhythm

Mu rhythm is not a common feature of normal EEGs. It is a run of negative wicket-shaped spikes with an approximate frequency of 10 Hz and a duration ranging from less than 1 second to many seconds. The negativity is maximal in the rolandic regions, mainly C3 and C4. Mu has the appearance of

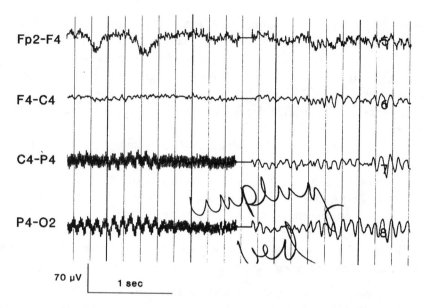

Figure 12.8   Machine artifact. The very high frequency artifact on the left side of the trace was from an air bed. Unplugging the bed abolished the artifact.

a centrally located alpha rhythm but is usually slightly faster than the patient's alpha rhythm. It is blocked by movement of the contralateral extremity, which is the key to identification. In fact, Mu may be blocked by merely thinking about limb movement. The technician should ask the patient to move a limb to verify the waveform.

Lambda Waves

Lambda waves are normal positive waves that appear over the occipital region when the patient is looking at a picture or pattern. Lambda waves indicate visual exploration and are blocked by eye closing. They are called lambda waves because of their resemblance to the Greek lowercase letter λ.

Wicket Spikes

Wicket spikes are sharply contoured waves that are most prominent in the temporal regions during drowsiness and light sleep. They are differentiated from true spikes by the absence of a following slow wave, normal background activity, and occurrence in trains at 6 to 10 per second. Wicket spikes are more common with increasing age.

"14 and 6" Hz Positive Spikes

The "14 and 6" Hz positive spike rhythm is a sharply contoured positive waveform that occurs mainly in drowsiness and light sleep. The distribution can be widespread but reaches highest amplitude over the posterior temporal region. At times, the rhythm has the appearance of 14 Hz, and at others it appears to be 6 Hz. Both frequencies may not occur together or in a particular patient during a single recording. The 6-Hz component predominates in young children and the 14-Hz frequency predominates in older children.

Although 14 and 6 positive spikes have been reported in association with many pathological conditions, the association is weak and the incidence is probably not different than in normal individuals. The 14-and-6 pattern should be described in the body of the EEG report but not interpreted as abnormal. One exception is in metabolic encephalopathies, such as hepatic coma. In this situation, the presence of 14 and 6 positive spikes is not considered normal but the background is abnormal as well.

Benign Epileptiform Transients of Sleep

Benign epileptiform transients of sleep (BETS) are very small spike-like potentials that occur in the temporal regions during drowsiness and light sleep. They are less than 50 μV with a duration of less than 15 ms. Also called "small sharp spikes," BETS are differentiated from epileptogenic spikes by their small amplitude, short duration, lack of slow wave, and normal EEG background.

Slow Alpha Variant

The slow alpha variant is a subharmonic of the normal alpha rhythm. The frequency is 4 to 5 Hz and the wave is usually notched, so that the native 10-Hz alpha rhythm can be identified.

Differentiation of the slow alpha variant from a diffuse encephalopathy is made by looking for the notching, and examining the background activity. Most conditions that would slow the posterior dominant rhythm to 4 to 5 Hz in an adult would be associated with a poorly organized background with theta anteriorly.

Rhythmic Temporal Theta of Drowsiness

Rhythmic temporal theta of drowsiness has been called the "psychomotor variant." This term should not be used because the implication is inappropriate. The rhythm consists of trains of sharply contoured waves in

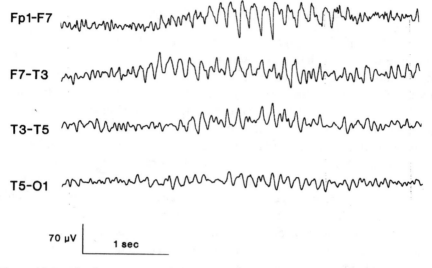

Figure 12.9 Rhythmic temporal theta of drowsiness.

the theta range (Figure 12.9). They are most prominent in the temporal region, but also present in central regions. As the name suggests, the rhythm is seen mainly in drowsiness, but may also be seen in relaxed wakefulness.

Rhythmic temporal theta of drowsiness is differentiated from seizure activity by the normal background before and after the train, and by the absence of typical frequency progression that characterizes most seizure discharges.

Mittens

Mittens are waveforms that are occasionally mistaken for spike-wave complexes. A sleep spindle and a vertex wave are partially fused, such that the last wave of the spindle is superimposed on the rising phase of the vertex wave. The voltage summation gives the last spindle wave a taller, faster appearance, simulating a spike. The name is derived from the appearance of a mitten; the thumb is the fused spindle wave, and the hand portion is the slow component of the vertex wave.

13 ⬚⬚⬚ ⬚⬚⬚ ⬚⬚⬚

Activation Methods

Activation methods are used to bring out epileptiform discharges in patients with suspected seizure disorders. Hyperventilation and photic stimulation are routinely used during EEG. Sleep is not considered by some neurophysiologists to be a true activation method, but certainly does aid in evoking epileptiform discharges.

Hyperventilation

The most predictable use of hyperventilation is to activate the three-per-second spike and wave discharge of primary generalized epilepsy. In some patients, discharges are only seen during hyperventilation. The patient is asked to mouth-breathe deeply for about three minutes. If there is suspicion of absence seizures, the patient should hyperventilate for five minutes.

The normal response to hyperventilation is generalized slowing of the background activity to the theta range in both hemispheres. Absence of slowing is not abnormal and depends in part on patient effort, age (children are more likely to show slowing than adults), and time from last meal (hypoglycemia may augment slowing). Movement artifact may contaminate the record, especially in the posterior leads, as a result of head movement with chest excursions. Normal slow activity may have a notched appearance and should not be interpreted as epileptiform. The epileptiform discharges activated by hyperventilation are usually not subtle.

Hyperventilation should not be performed in patients with cerebrovascular disease or intracranial hemorrhage. Hypocapnia and alkalosis may cause vasospasm and impair cerebral perfusion.

The mechanism by which hyperventilation activates epileptiform activity is not completely known. The effect of hyperventilation-induced alkalosis and hypocapnia on the caliber of cerebral vessels is probably not important in the genesis of epileptiform discharges. The development of slow activity and disinhibition of spikes and slow waves may be due to depression of activity of the reticular activating system.

Photic Stimulation

Photic stimulation is more likely to activate epileptiform discharges in patients with primary rather than secondary epilepsy. A strobe light is placed in front of the patient's closed eyes. The light delivers trains of flashes at specified rates. These routines are programmed into most EEG machines. General guidelines for performing photic stimulation are:

1. Train duration = 10 sec.
2. Trains delivered every 20 sec.
3. Initial flash rate of 3/sec.
4. Each successive train has a higher frequency. For example, we use the following flash rates in our laboratory: 3, 5, 7, 9, 11, 13, 15, 18, 20, 24, 30 per second.
5. If a discharge is activated at a specified frequency, the technician should repeat that frequency at the completion of the photic stimulation routine.

Normal responses to photic stimulation include the visual evoked response, the driving response, and the photomyoclonic response.

Normal Photic Response

A visual evoked response can be seen in occipital leads at flash frequencies less than 7/sec (Figure 13.1). This response is the same as the flash-induced visual evoked potential discussed in chapter 31, "Visual Evoked Potential," but is much more variable because the response is not averaged. A driving response is seen at flash frequencies of 7/sec and greater (Figure 13.2). The two responses look alike but are distinguished by their temporal relation to the stimulus. The visual evoked response occurs approximately 100 ms after the stimulus, and the driving response is exactly time-locked to the stimulus.

The absence of visual evoked and driving responses is not abnormal unless it is well developed on one side and absent on the other. Such asymmetry suggests an abnormality affecting either the projections from the lateral geniculate to the cortex or the calcarine cortex itself.

Photomyoclonic Response

The photomyoclonic response is caused by repeated contraction of frontal muscles that are time-locked to the flash stimulus. Muscle activity (EMG) that may have the appearance of seizure discharges appears in the anterior leads. Factors that help distinguish a photomyoclonic response from a photoconvulsive discharge are:

1. The photomyoclonic response is anterior, while photoconvulsive responses are posterior or generalized.

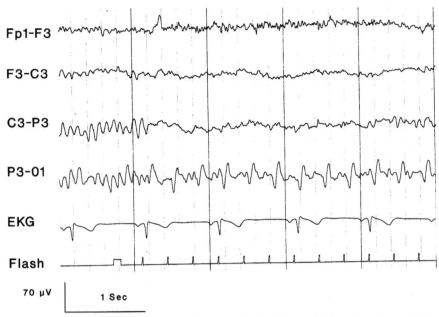

Figure 13.1 Photic evoked potential. Note the lag between the stimulus and the peak of the evoked potential in channel 4. This lag plus the response only at low frequencies differentiates the evoked response from the driving response.

2. The photomyoclonic response stops promptly at the end of the stimulus train, while the photoconvulsive response typically outlasts the stimulus.
3. The "spikes" that make up the photomyoclonic response are much faster than those of cerebral origin. The synchrony of muscle fiber discharges is much greater than that of neuronal discharges.

The photomyoclonic response is enhanced in patients undergoing alcohol or barbiturate withdrawal and should be considered as a nonspecific, normal response despite unconfirmed reports of an association with seizures and psychiatric disorders.

Photoconvulsive Response

The photoconvulsive response is characterized by spike-wave complexes during photic stimulation (Figure 13.3). The discharge is usually activated only by a few specific flash frequencies. It never begins with the first flash, and usually ends before the flash ends. The correlation of a photoconvulsive discharge with seizures is greatest if the discharges continue after the end of flash train.

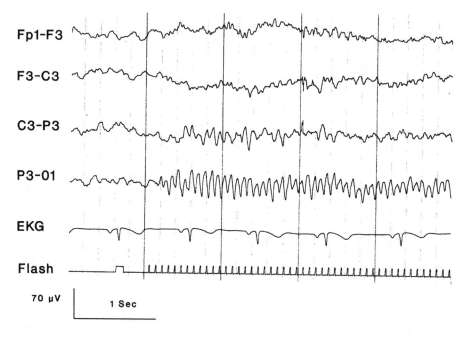

Figure 13.2 Photic driving response. The driving response is time-locked to the flash, without the lag that characterizes the evoked response. Also, the driving response is present at faster frequencies.

Sleep

The frequency of interictal epileptiform discharges is often increased during drowsiness and light sleep. Therefore, patients being evaluated for a seizure disorder should be studied both when awake and when asleep.

Sleep is also helpful to identify potentials that are seen in the waking state. For example, subtle sharp transients may be evident in the waking state which are not clearly epileptiform. During sleep, the spikes may be activated into definite epileptiform activity. Conversely, sharp transients that disappear during sleep are unlikely to be epileptiform. They may be normal waveforms with unusually sharp contours or artifact.

Since most routine EEG recordings are performed in the waking state, sedation or sleep deprivation is often necessary. There is no convincing evidence that spontaneous sleep, sedated sleep, and sleep by deprivation differ in their ability to evoke epileptiform activity.

Sedated Sleep

Chloral hydrate is commonly used for sedation because it is safe to use in outpatients and does not produce the widespread beta activity that is characteristic of benzodiazepines and barbiturates. The usual oral dose for

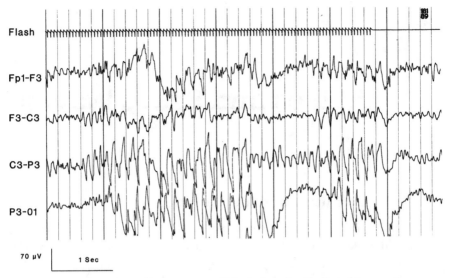

Figure 13.3   Photoconvulsive response. Note that the discharge is not time-locked to the stimulus and outlasts the train of flashes.

adults is 1 gm, with a single repeat if needed. Children receive 25 mg/kg; this may be repeated up to 75 mg/kg. The major side effects of chloral hydrate in adults are confusion and ataxia. Therefore, all outpatients who are sedated must have an attendant who will look after them and drive them home. Children can have confusion and ataxia, but may alternatively develop an agitated delirium.

Barbiturates are an alternative to chloral hydrate and are especially useful in patients with a history of chloral hydrate agitation. Intravenous administration of short-acting barbiturates has been advocated by some investigators for the detection of focal epileptiform activity; however, this is not routine practice.

Sleep Deprivation

Sleep deprivation entails keeping the patient awake for twenty-four hours prior to the recording. After arising one day, the patient does not sleep until the EEG is performed the following morning. The patient is discouraged from drinking caffeine-containing beverages. Patients who adhere to the sleep deprivation regimen usually fall asleep during the recording. Unfortunately, patients often progress quickly into stage 3 or 4 sleep, missing the transition from wakefulness through drowsiness into light sleep. This progression is most important for detection of spikes. Therefore, it is helpful to keep the patient awake and watch the drowsy pattern for epileptiform activity. Sleep deprivation for twenty-four hours does not evoke spikes in normal individuals. Therefore, concern over false positives is unfounded.

14 □ □ □
□ □ □
□ □ □

Spikes and Sharp Waves

Definition and Identification

Spikes and sharp waves are transients that stand out from the background. Spikes are usually surface negative and have a duration of 20 to 70 ms. Sharp waves are also usually surface negative but have a duration of 70 to 200 ms. Pointed potentials with a duration of less than 20 ms are usually not of cerebral origin. The negative pole of spikes and sharp waves is distributed across a region of the cortex. The distribution is called a *potential field.* This field is not directly comparable to the field potential recorded by intracortical electrodes. The positive end of the spike dipole is occasionally visible on the surface, usually indicating that the dipole is oriented horizontally.

Table 14.1 lists criteria for differentiating spikes from nonspike potentials. Major pitfalls include misinterpreting sharply contoured slow waves and pointed waves of background rhythms. Theta activity occurs normally in drowsiness and in children. The theta is polymorphic and multiple waves occasionally sum to give a sharp appearance. A sharp wave should not be considered abnormal unless it stands out from the background and is reproducible. The alpha rhythm may occasionally appear sharp, even though the pointed component is positive. Positive polarity helps to distinguish this waveform from a spike potential. The sharp component occurs in step with the other waves comprising the alpha rhythm, indicating that it is merely a sharply contoured alpha wave and not a pathological spike.

In general, more harm is done by overinterpretation than by underinterpretation of electroencephalography (EEG). If you are uncertain that a potential is abnormal, consider it to be normal. The questionable potential should be described in the body of the report to facilitate comparison with future studies.

When spike potentials are seen in studies requested for nonseizure indications, it is not helpful to interpret the record as "consistent with a seizure disorder." Instead, interpret the record as follows: "This is an abnormal study because of a spike focus in the left posterior temporal region. Spikes are not always associated with a seizure disorder."

Table 14.1   Differentiation between Spike and Nonspike Potentials

Spike	Nonspike
Stereotyped	Vary in morphology
Stand out from the background	Embedded in the background
Rising phase is fastest	May be slower rising phase than spike
Usually a following slow wave	Usually no slow wave
Defined potential field	Often a single electrode
Activated by sleep	No change with sleep

Note: In addition to this differentiation, it is important to distinguish pathological from nonpathological sharp waveforms, especially normal sharp waves in neonates, vertex waves, lambda waves, 14 and 6 positive spikes, mu rhythm, and artifacts.

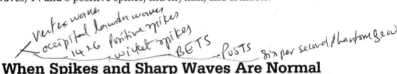

When Spikes and Sharp Waves Are Normal

Most spikes and sharp waves are abnormal in adults. However, several physiological spike-like potentials may be recorded. These include vertex waves, occipital lambda waves, 14 and 6 positive spikes, wicket spikes, benign epileptiform transients of sleep (BETS), positive occipital sharp transients of sleep (POSTS), and six-per-second phantom spike and wave. These are discussed in chapter 12, "Normal Electroencephalography Patterns."

Normal infants occasionally exhibit frontal or temporal sharp waves. Guidelines for distinguishing normal from pathological sharp waves are presented in chapter 17, "Neonatal Electroencephalography."

Generalized Spike-wave Discharge

Spike and wave complexes correlate better than single spike discharges with clinical seizures. Generalized spike-wave discharges fall into four categories: three-per-second spike and wave, slow spike-wave complex, fast spike-wave complex, and six-per-second spike wave.

Three-per-Second Spike-wave Complex

The three-per-second (3/sec) spike-wave complex is usually equated with absence seizures. While there is a strong correlation between the two, a patient with 3/sec spike-wave complex may exhibit other seizure types, including generalized tonic-clonic seizures. The interpretation of such records should read: "Abnormal study because of 3/sec spike-wave complexes. This is consistent with a seizure disorder of the generalized type."

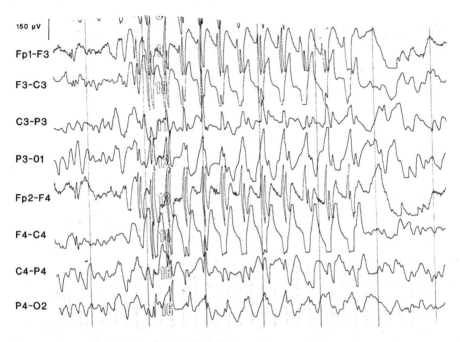

Figure 14.1   Three-per-second spike wave complex. Typical discharge occurring during hyperventilation. Multiple episodes occurred during the recording.

Characteristics of the Three-per-Second Spike-wave Complex

The 3/sec spike-wave complex is synchronous from the two hemispheres, with highest amplitude over the midline frontal region. The lowest amplitudes are in the temporal and occipital regions. The frequency changes slightly during the course of the discharge, beginning close to 4/sec and declining to 2.5/sec. Immediately following the discharge, the record quickly returns to normal (Figure 14.1). The spike component may have a double spike or polyspike appearance.

The 3/sec spike-wave complex is promoted by hyperventilation. If absence epilepsy is considered, the patient should be asked to hyperventilate for five minutes instead of the usual three minutes. Children with absence become symptomatic if the discharge lasts longer than five seconds. During the discharge, the technician should ask the child a question. The child with absence often answers after the discharge. The question and response should be noted on the record.

The 3/sec discharge is less well organized during sleep than during the waking state. Its appearance is more polyspike in configuration and the spike-wave interval is less regular.

Occasional patients with typical 3/sec spike-wave complex have small amplitude frontal spikes called *fragments*. These can be asymmetric, but are seen from both hemispheres. The implication of fragments is controversial. They should be mentioned in the body of the report but should not change the final impression.

Clinical Correlations of the Three-per-Second Spike-wave Complex

The 3/sec spike-wave discharge correlates well with primary generalized epilepsy. Factors that should make the clinician doubt the diagnosis of primary generalized epilepsy include (1) abnormal background on the EEG, (2) clearly focal discharges, or (3) history of slow development or an abnormal neurologic examination.

The spike component of the 3/sec complex is polyspike in some patients with absence epilepsy. Patients with this polyspike pattern are more likely to exhibit myoclonus.

Treatment of absence epilepsy abolishes the interictal discharge. This is different from most focal epilepsies, where interictal spiking persists despite good seizure control.

Slow Spike-wave Complex

The slow spike-wave complex is frequently associated clinically with the Lennox-Gastaut syndrome. It also has been called the "petit mal variant." The term is misleading and should not be used.

The frequency of the slow spike-wave complex is 2.5/sec or less, and its morphology is less stereotyped than the 3/sec complex. The duration of the slow spike is usually more than 70 ms, technically a sharp wave. The complex is generalized, synchronous across both hemispheres, and with highest amplitude in the midline frontal region.

During sleep, the slow spike-wave activity may be continuous. This may not indicate status epilepticus but is rather activation of the interictal pattern with sleep.

Lennox-Gastaut Syndrome

The slow spike-wave complex is usually an interictal pattern but may be ictal as well. Since these patients have a mixed seizure disorder, ictal events may be characterized by patterns other than the slow spike-wave complex.

Atonic seizures are characterized by generalized spikes during the myoclonus, followed by the slow spike-wave pattern during the atonic phase. Atonic seizures are most characteristic of the Lennox-Gastaut syndrome.

Akinetic seizures are characterized by the slow spike-wave discharge throughout the seizure. Tonic seizures also occur in Lennox-Gastaut syn-

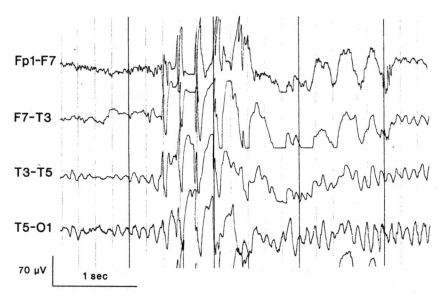

Fp1-F7

F7-T3

T3-T5

T5-O1

70 µV   1 sec

Figure 14.2   Fast spike wave complex in a patient with juvenile myoclonic epilepsy.

drome and are characterized rapid spike activity or desynchronization rather than the slow spike-wave pattern.

Fast Spike-wave Complex

The fast spike-wave complex has a frequency of 4 to 5/sec and is characterized by generalized spikes followed by slow waves (Figure 14.2). Maximal amplitude is in the fronto-central region. Patients have generalized tonic-clonic seizures with or without myoclonus. Absence seizures are rare. This is the most common pattern seen in patients with idiopathic generalized tonic-clonic seizures. The discharge is not as stereotyped and synchronous as the 3/sec spike-wave complex.

Six-per-Second Hz (Phantom) Spike-wave Complex

The six-per-second (6/sec) phantom spike and wave pattern is characterized by brief trains of small spike and wave complexes that are distributed diffusely over both hemispheres. They are most common during the waking and drowsy states, and disappear during sleep.

The 6/sec spike-wave complex may have frontal or occipital predominance. Frontal predominance is frequently associated with generalized tonic-clonic seizures, while occipital predominance is usually not associated with clinical seizures. Hughes (1980) provided the acronyms, WHAM and FOLD. WHAM stands for *w*aking record, *h*igh amplitude, *a*nterior, *m*ales; FOLD for *f*emales, *o*ccipital, *l*ow amplitude, *d*rowsy. WHAM is associated with seizures; FOLD is not.

This rhythm is differentiated from the 14- and 6-Hz positive spikes not only by the polarity, but also by the more widespread distribution, and occurrence in wakefulness. Both rhythms may occur in the same patient. The 6/sec spike-wave complex is interpreted as abnormal and the different clinical implications should be emphasized in the report.

Hypsarrhythmia

Hypsarrhythmia is seen in children with infantile spasms. High-voltage bursts of theta and delta waves have multifocal sharp waves superimposed (Figure 14.3). The bursts are separated by periods of relative suppression. In some circumstances, flattening of the EEG may be an ictal sign, indicating that there has been sudden desynchronization of the record.

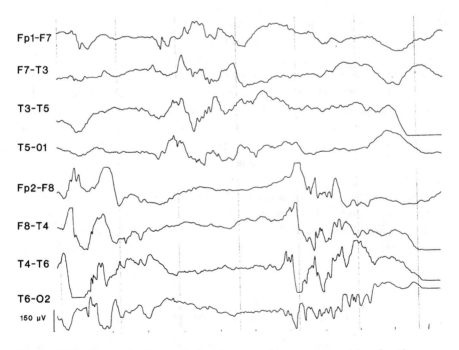

Figure 14.3 Hypsarrhythmia. A sleeping record in a patient with infantile spasms. During the waking state the periods of suppression are not as prominent.

Focal Spikes

Focal spikes often indicate a focal seizure disorder. Fronto-central discharges may be seen in patients with simple partial seizures. Temporal or frontal spikes may be seen in patients with complex partial seizures. Normal focal spike-wave complexes include 14 and 6 positive spikes, rhythmic temporal theta of drowsiness, subclinical rhythmic EEG discharge of adults, and wicket spikes.

Focal spikes are only diagnosed if the spike is consistent, has a definable field, and cannot be explained by artifact. A single spike during the course of a recording should not be interpreted as abnormal. Also, great caution should be exercised when interpreting a spike that is only seen from a single electrode (remember that a single electrode may be represented on more than one channel in a montage).

Focal Spikes Associated with Epilepsy

Focal spikes are associated with partial seizures and the benign epilepsies of childhood. Partial seizures are subdivided into simple and complex, based on the symptomatology. Benign epilepsies of childhood are associated with focal and generalized seizures.

During simple partial seizures, the EEG usually shows prominent spiking over the involved cortex, but in some patients there is localized slowing that may become generalized. A typical pattern would be left-central spikes in a patient who presents with focal seizures affecting the right arm. Occasionally, the sharp component of the discharge may be subtle or missing altogether. The epileptiform activity may occur in deep layers of cortex and subcortical structures, so that the spike potentials are not projected to surface electrodes. Alternatively, there may not be sufficient synchrony to produce a spike detectable on the surface.

During complex partial seizures, the EEG usually shows focal spikes in the temporal or frontal region. Routine EEG may not detect the spikes if they originate in cortex that is not directly underlying the surface electrodes. Sphenoidal, nasopharyngeal, or depth electrodes may be needed to identify these discharges.

Benign Focal Epilepsies of Childhood

Benign focal epilepsies of childhood are termed *benign* because they are age-related and do not persist into adult life. There are two types: rolandic and occipital.

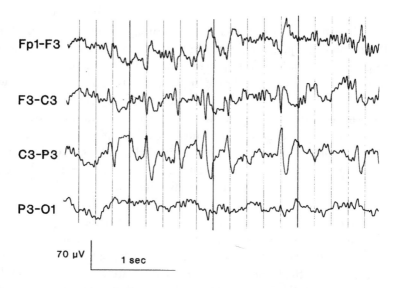

Fp1-F3

F3-C3

C3-P3

P3-O1

70 µV | 1 sec

Figure 14.4 Central spikes in a patient with rolandic epilepsy.

Rolandic Epilepsy

Rolandic epilepsy is characterized by interictal independent focal discharges in the central regions, predominantly C3 and C4, that are augmented during sleep. Relatives of patients with rolandic epilepsy may have the EEG abnormality as a genetic marker without clinical seizures.

The discharges of rolandic epilepsy are so characteristic that they are seldom confused with other patterns (Figure 14.4). Independent central spikes are seen on an otherwise normal background. However, this must be differentiated from multifocal spikes.

Occipital Epilepsy

Occipital epilepsy is characterized by interictal sharp waves with predominance at O1 and O2. Rolandic and occipital epilepsy may occur in the same families, and relatives with no history of seizures may have either occipital or rolandic discharges on EEG.

During the seizure, the EEG shows 2 to 3/sec spike-wave discharges with predominance in the occipital region. The interictal discharge may be blocked by photic stimulation or by eye opening.

Focal Sharp Waves without Clinical Seizures

Patients with no clinical evidence of seizure activity are occasionally found to have focal spikes or sharp waves. Some of these are children who are genetic carriers of benign focal epilepsies; in others there is no explanation. The interpretation of these records is controversial. Some electroencephalographers believe that all sharp activity is potentially epileptogenic and should be interpreted as such. Unfortunately, this may result in unneeded use of antiepileptic drugs. Patients should be treated with antiepileptic drugs based on clinical presentation rather than on EEG findings. The old adage is still valid: "Treat the patient. Do not treat the EEG."

Approximately 3% of normal individuals exhibit epileptiform activity on EEG. The proportion is somewhat higher in children than adults. Approximately 25% of these discharges are focal. Some of these patients will go on to develop seizures; however, the patients should not be treated with anticonvulsants without clinical evidence of convulsive activity.

Children with behavioral disturbances have been reported to have an increased incidence of focal sharp waves and spikes. The implication of these waveforms is controversial. Some investigators believe that the spikes may have contributed to the behavioral disturbance by interfering with normal social and intellectual development. Others believe that the spikes are incidental and should not be treated. The spikes are probably a reflection of brain dysfunction, which correlates with the behavioral disorder rather than being the cause of the disturbance.

Subclinical rhythmic EEG discharge of adults (SREDA) is sharply contoured rhythmic theta activity with prominence in the centro-parietal region. This pattern is seen in older patients and has no definite clinical correlate. This is not an ictal discharge. Patients with this finding are said to be at increased risk for cerebrovascular disease, but the association is not convincing (Miller et al. 1985). This rhythm is not found in normal younger individuals and is probably an abnormal pattern. However, the report should reflect the nonspecific clinical implications.

Some patients with congenital blindness may exhibit occipital spikes. These should not be interpreted as epileptiform.

Periodic Patterns

Periodic Lateralized Epileptiform Discharges

Periodic lateralized epileptiform discharges (PLEDs) are high-amplitude sharp waves that recur at a rate of 0.5 to 3/sec (Figure 14.5). They are prominent over one hemisphere or one region. When bilateral, they are independent, thereby keeping the term lateralized.

A sign of parenchymal destruction, PLEDs are most often seen in strokes, but are also seen with head injury, abscess, encephalitis, hypoxic encephalopathy, brain tumors, and other focal lesions. It is impossible to distinguish definitively between causations on the basis of waveform. Of the

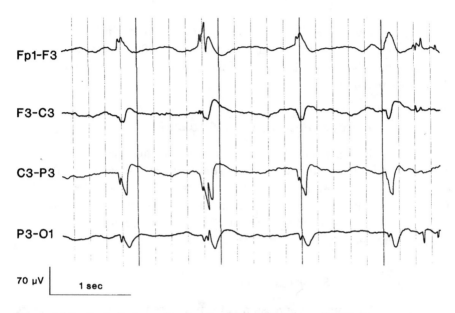

Figure 14.5 Periodic lateralized epileptiform discharges (PLEDs) in a patient with hypoxic encephalopathy. The contralateral side showed a similar pattern, although there was no synchrony between the hemispheres.

encephalitides, herpes simplex most commonly produces PLEDs. Other viral infections produce slowing without PLEDs.

The PLEDs have an amplitude of 100 to 300 μV. An early negative component is followed by a positive wave. The discharge may be complex, with additional sharp and slow components superimposed on the waveform.

Patients with PLEDs may have myoclonic jerks that are either synchronous with the PLEDs or independent. When the jerks are independent, the generator for the myoclonus is probably deep. Even when they are synchronous, the generator is probably subcortical. The cortical discharge reflects projections from the deep generator.

Periodic Pattern with Herpes Simplex Encephalitis

The EEG usually shows PLEDs at some time in the course of herpes simplex encephalitis. Initially, there may be only slow activity in the theta and, subsequently, in the delta range. The PLEDs are sharply contoured slow waves with a frequency of 2 to 4 Hz. The duration of each wave is often more than 50 ms. This relatively slow frequency of repetition helps to differentiate PLEDs in herpes encephalitis from the higher frequency discharges of subacute sclerosing panencephalitis.

Neonates with herpes encephalitis may have necrosis that is not confined or even most prominent in the temporal region. Also, PLEDs may not be seen. The EEG may show a poorly organized background with slow activity in the delta range predominating.

Periodic Pattern with Anoxic Encephalopathy

Patients with hypoxic-ischemic encephalopathy have disorganization of the background with diffuse slowing and suppression. Periodic sharp waves are often seen, and may predominate in the record. They look like PLEDs, except that they are synchronous between hemispheres. Patients may have myoclonus associated with the discharges. These probably represent an extreme of the burst suppression pattern.

Burst Suppression

The burst-suppression pattern occurs in patients with severe encephalopathies. The finding is not specific as to etiology but is most often seen in patients with hypoxic-ischemic damage and in barbiturate coma.

The burst-suppression pattern seen in patients in barbiturate coma is very similar to that seen in the twenty-nine-week gestation newborn. Bursts of slow waves with superimposed sharp activity are superimposed upon a very suppressed background. The background is not flat, but rather is very low voltage, composed of a mixture of frequencies. Barbiturate coma is used to protect the brain in patients with serious central nervous system insults, such as head injuries and intractable seizures.

Periodic Pattern with Subacute Sclerosing Panencephalitis

Subacute sclerosing panencephalitis (SSPE) has almost disappeared as a result of mass measles immunization. Periodic complexes are seen in most patients at an intermediate stage. Early on, there may be only mild slowing with disorganization of the background. Late in the course, the periodic complexes may completely disappear, leaving the recording virtually isoelectric. The discharges are slow waves with sharp components. The duration of the complex is up to 3 seconds, and the interval between complexes is 5 to 15 seconds. The background during the interval is disorganized and generally suppressed. Myoclonus is typically synchronous with the discharge.

The EEG in SSPE closely resembles that of burst suppression. The background is usually more suppressed with burst suppression than in SSPE. The two patterns are more easily differentiated by clinical presentation. Patients with burst suppression usually have a known history of hypoxia or severe metabolic derangement. They also have a typical history of a progressive neurologic disorder characterized by intellectual deterioration and seizures. Subacute sclerosing panencephalitis is very rare.

Periodic Pattern with Jakob-Creutzfeld Disease

Jakob-Creutzfeld disease is characterized by periodic complexes composed of a sharp wave or sharply contoured slow wave. The interval between discharges is 500 to 2,000 ms. The discharges are maximal in the anterior regions and may occasionally be unilateral. Only rarely are the discharges predominant posteriorally, and then they are commonly associated with blindness. The discharges may or may not be temporally locked to myoclonus. These discharges are superimposed on an abnormal background, characterized by low-voltage slowing in the theta and delta range. The periodic complexes disappear during sleep.

15 ⬜⬜⬜ ⬜⬜⬜ ⬜⬜⬜

Slow Activity

Slowing may be generalized or focal. Generalized slow activity usually indicates encephalopathy. Focal slow activity usually indicates a structural lesion.

Generalized Slowing

Slowing of the Posterior Dominant Rhythm

A posterior dominant rhythm of less than 8.5 Hz is always abnormal in adults. Such slowing is usually bilateral, and is often interpreted as indicating a diffuse encephalopathy. Bilateral occipital lesions may also result in loss of the posterior alpha rhythm. These lesions may result in cortical blindness. Figure 15.1 shows focal slowing superimposed upon a generalized slow background.

Slow Activity Superimposed on the Waking Background

Theta and delta activity in waking records are usually abnormal. An important exception is the occipital delta of posterior slow waves of youth, discussed in chapter 12, "Normal Electroencephalography Patterns." Waking records contain a small amount of theta, but this is usually overshadowed by alpha and faster frequencies. Patients with low-voltage records may seem to have excessive theta if the gain is increased, but at a normal gain of 7 μV/mm, the theta is not prominent.

Generalized Slowing in Sleep Recordings

Electroencephalographic (EEG) frequencies during sleep are generally slower than in the waking state. The activity is very slow during the deeper stages of sleep (3 and 4) with virtual abolition of normal fast frequencies. These deep-sleep stages may be misinterpreted as an encephalopathy.

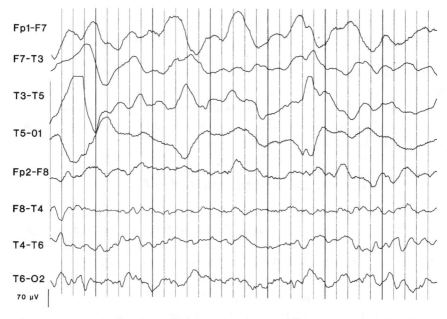

Figure 15.1 Generalized and focal slowing. The record shows slowing most prominent from the left hemisphere, although both hemispheres were slow.

Encephalopathy should be diagnosed during sleep only if the background is nonreactive and incompatible with any stage of the sleep cycle. Even then, a waking record should be examined if at all possible.

Conversely, normal sleeping EEG activity does not rule out an encephalopathy. It is possible to have abnormal slowing during the waking state and normal sleep patterns. Therefore, the diagnosis of encephalopathy cannot be excluded if only a normal sleeping record is provided. The EEG report should reflect these limitations on interpretation of encephalopathy in the sleeping state. The report might read, "Normal sleeping EEG. Encephalopathy is difficult to diagnose in the sleeping state. A waking record should be made if clinically indicated."

Focal Slowing

Focal slowing usually correlates with focal structural lesions of the hemispheres. The slowing usually overlies the lesion, but does not always correlate precisely. The slowing is irregular and composed of delta activity with theta superimposed. It is termed *polymorphic delta activity* (PDA) because of the variability in waveform morphology. Faster frequencies meld with the slow activity. For reasons that are unclear, PDA may not be continuous, but instead may punctuate an otherwise normal EEG background.

The neurophysiological substrate of PDA is not understood completely. In general, PDA is interpreted as being due to an abnormality in the white-matter relays between the cortex and subcortical nuclei.

Polymorphic delta activity is the most common finding in focal structural lesions such as tumors, contusion, hemorrhage, infarction, and abscess. Focal spikes or sharp waves without another disturbance of the background is seldom a sign of a focal parenchymal lesion. Focal slowing is nonspecific; there are no characteristics that distinguish one cause from another.

Intermittent Rhythmic Delta Activity

Intermittent rhythmic delta activity is always a sign of cerebral dysfunction. The distribution across the hemispheres depends on the age of the patient. In adults, the activity is predominantly frontal—frontal intermittent rhythmic delta activity (FIRDA). In children, the activity is more commonly posterior—posterior intermittent rhythmic delta activity (PIRDA) or occipital intermittent rhythmic delta activity (OIRDA).

Intermittent rhythmic delta activity is thought to be caused by a disconnection of activity between the deep nuclei and cerebral cortex. This EEG pattern should be interpreted as showing cerebral dysfunction without implications for localization. There are no diagnostic differences between FIRDA and PIRDA.

Seizures Manifest as Rhythmic Slow Waves

Seizures may occasionally be manifest on routine EEG as rhythmic slow waves. Presumably, the spike component is either very small in amplitude or not projected to the cortical surface.

Differentiating epileptiform slow waves from FIRDA, PIRDA, or PDA may be difficult. Epileptiform slow activity interferes with the normal background, while FIRDA may be associated with an otherwise near-normal background. Epileptiform slow activity is differentiated from PDA by the stereotypic nature of the epileptiform activity. The waves tend to be smoother, and if the discharges are bilateral, there is usually a high degree of interhemispheric synchrony.

Focal Loss of Electroencephalographic Patterns

Focal attenuation of EEG activity, especially loss of beta activity, usually indicates a structural lesion. Occipital lesions may cause unilateral loss of the posterior alpha. Unilateral lesions may also disrupt sleep patterns so that sleep spindles and/or vertex waves are not seen from the affected hemisphere.

16

Cerebral Death Studies

Guidelines for Determination of Brain Death

The guidelines for determination of brain death are based on the consensus of the president's commission (Medical Consultants on the Diagnosis of Death 1981). For brain death, the patient must meet the following criteria:

- Cessation of all brain functions
- Recovery not possible
- Cause of coma known.

Clinical examination for cerebral death should show the following findings:

- No pupillary reflexes
- No corneal responses
- No response to auditory or visual stimuli
- No response to "doll's head maneuver"
- No response to ice water calorics
- No respiratory efforts with apnea testing.

The clinician must ensure that the absence of responsiveness is not due to drug intoxication, metabolic disturbance, or neuromuscular blockade. Therefore, the following should be ensured:

- Temperature ≥ 90°F
- Systolic blood pressure ≥ 80 mm Hg
- No toxic levels of central nervous system depressants
- No neuromuscular blockade.

Patients being evaluated for brain death will frequently be hypothermic and hypotensive; therefore, maintenance on warming blankets and pressors is often required. The presence of tendon reflexes argues against neuromuscular blockade.

The guidelines for determination of cerebral death indicate that there should be a period of observation, with documentation of examinations for cerebral death before and after this period. If the cause of coma is not anoxia, the period of observation must be twelve hours. If the cause is anoxia, the period of observation is twenty-four hours.

This period of observation can be shortened if there is a confirmatory test. These include:

- Electroencephalography (EEG)
- Brainstem auditory evoked potential
- Radionucleotide flow study
- Angiogram.

Recently, transcranial doppler has been studied as a confirmatory test for brain death. Since brain death is a complex legal issue, and the president's commission did not specifically mention transcranial doppler, this technique should not be used until the clinician can be assured that this is accepted medical practice.

In general, cerebral death should be established on the basis of clinical findings alone. Some patients with no clinical evidence of cerebral or brainstem activity will have evidence of EEG activity but otherwise fulfill the clinical criteria for brain death. The literature is not clear on what to do in this situation. The probability of meaningful neurologic recovery is virtually nonexistent if the patient has no evidence of cerebral or brainstem function throughout an appropriate period of observation, regardless of the results of a confirmatory test.

Guidelines for Brain Death in Children

The 1981 president's commission did not make specific recommendations for determination of brain death in children. The only specific comment recommended "caution in children under the age of five years." A task force for brain death in children subsequently provided recommendations that are increasingly used. The recommendations follow those outlined for adults above except as follows:

1. Do not declare a patient under the age of 7 days brain dead. Clinical and EEG criteria are not established for this early period.
2. Between 7 days and 2 months of age, perform two examinations and two EEGs forty-eight hours apart.
3. Between 2 months and 1 year of age, perform two examinations and two EEGs twenty-four hours apart.
4. Above 1 year of age, perform two examinations twelve hours apart without a confirmatory test. The observation period can be six hours if a single EEG is done.

Despite these recommendations, most pediatricians do not feel comfortable declaring brain death without a confirmatory test.

Electroencephalography for Cerebral Death

Technical standards for the determination of cerebral death include the following recommendations:

1. Minimum of eight scalp electrodes covering all brain regions. This is usually a reduced version of the 10-20 Electrode Placement System. The following electrodes are recommended as a minimum: Fp1, Fp2, C3, C4, O1, O2, T3, T4.
2. Interelectrode distances of at least 10 cm. This allows for better detection of low-amplitude EEG activity. A minimal montage would be:

Channel No.	Montage
1	Fp1-C3
2	C3-O1
3	Fp2-C4
4	C4-O2
5	Fp1-T3
6	T3-O1
7	Fp2-T4
8	T4-O2

3. Interelectrode impedances no greater than 10 kohms, but less than 100 ohms. Too low an impedance occurs with electrode-gel smear. The amplitude of recorded electrocerebral activity will be excessively low if the impedance is low.
4. Sensitivity of 2 µV/mm during most of the recording.
5. Time constant of 0.3–0.4 sec.
6. EKG monitoring and other physiological monitoring if necessary. Monitoring of chest-wall motion may be needed if there is apparent slow activity in the record.
7. Reactivity of the EEG tested to auditory, visual, and tactile stimuli.
8. Recording time of at least thirty minutes. Only include relatively artifact-free time.
9. Integrity of the system tested. Touching of the electrodes produces high-amplitude artifact on the EEG recording, ensuring that failure to detect activity is not due to technical problems.
10. Recording made by a qualified technologist.

Cerebral Death Studies in Adults

Cerebral death (CD) studies should be performed in the period of observation, between the two extensive neurological examinations. All of the above recommendations should be followed, but in addition, all of the physiological parameters set forth by the president's commission should be followed: (1) blood pressure at least 80-mm Hg systolic, (2) temperature of 90°F or greater, and (3) no sedatives.

Cerebral Death Studies in Children

Cerebral death studies in children are performed in the same manner as CD studies in adults. More physiological monitoring is often required than for adult studies. Because of small body size, respiratory movement artifact is relatively greater and a chest-wall sensor is desirable. An electrocardiogram (EKG) channel is desirable for adult CD studies, but is even more important for CD studies in children. At high sensitivities, EKG artifact is the predominant potential in the record.

17

□ □ □
□ □ □
□ □ □

Neonatal Electroencephalography

Technical Requirements

Recording Procedures

Neonatal electroencephalography (EEG) must be performed according to the guidelines for routine EEG in adults and children outlined in chapter 10. The sensitivities and filter settings are the same as those used for adult EEGs. At the initial sensitivity of 7 µV/mm, pen excursion is usually excessive and sensitivity reduction is needed.

The *Guidelines* recommend that at least three physiological parameters be monitored: respirations, eye movements, and electrocardiogram. Respirations can be rapid and produce an artifact that mimics slow activity in the EEG. Electrocardiogram (EKG) monitoring is useful to identify EKG and pulse artifacts. Eye-movement recordings and submental electromyography (EMG) help to identify wake and sleep states. These parameters are measured using procedures described in chapter 12, "Normal Electroencephalography Patterns."

Newborns spend most of their day sleeping and sedation is usually not required. The electrodes should be placed before the baby is fed. Most newborns fall asleep immediately after a feed. The newborn should be aroused during the study in order to observe arousal and the waking state.

Electrode impedance must be less than 10 kohm. The absolute impedance is not as important as consistency between impedances. If impedances are greater than 5 k, impedance checks for mismatch should be performed.

Photic stimulation is of no benefit in newborns. Driving responses are not reproducible and photoconvulsive discharges do not occur at this age. Hyperventilation is not performed.

Montages

A recommended montage for newborns includes a truncated version of the adult longitudinal bipolar montage plus several physiological

Table 17.1   Recommended Montages for Neonatal Electroencephalogram

Channel No.	LB	Ref	NB
1	Fp1-F3	Fp1-A1	Fp1-C3
2	F3-C3	Fp2-A2	C3-O1
3	C3-P3	F3-A1	Fp1-T3
4	Fp2-F4	F4-A2	T3-O1
5	C4-C4	C3-A1	Fp2-C4
6	C4-P4	C4-A2	C4-O2
7	F7-T3	P3-A1	Fp2-T4
8	T3-T5	P4-A4	T4-O2
9	T5-O1	O1-A1	T3-C3
10	F8-T4	O2-A2	C3-Cz
11	T4-T6	T3-A1	Cz-C4
12	T6-O2	T4-A2	C4-T4
13	EKG	EKG	EKG
14	Resp	Resp	Resp
15	Left EOM	Left EOM	Left EOM
16	Right EOM	Right EOM	Right EOM

LB = Longitudinal bipolar; Ref = Ear reference; NB = Newborn montage; EOM = Extra ocular movement.

Note: NB differs from LB in that there are double electrode distances and one channel includes vertex derivations.

Source: Recommendations are from American Electroencephalographic Society 1986.

functions (see Table 17.1). If fewer non-EEG channels are required, the bipolar montage may be more complete. The full longitudinal bipolar (LB) montage can be used if the recording is made using a twenty-one-channel machine. However, the placement of many electrodes on a small head increases the chance for electrode-gel smear with electrical contact between electrodes. Therefore, the truncated version of the LB montage is considered sufficient. Only one montage is recorded for the entire study.

Guidelines for Interpretation of Neonatal Electroencephalography

Accurate interpretation of neonatal EEG requires knowledge of the newborn's gestational age, postnatal age, physiological state, and reactivity. Conceptional age is the sum of gestational age and postnatal age. A term newborn is at least 38-weeks gestational age. Younger newborns are premature. The gestational, postnatal, and conceptional ages should be indicated on all neonatal EEG recordings.

Neonatal EEG is unfamiliar to most adult neurologists but is facilitated by the following guidelines:

1. Examine the frequency composition and distribution of the background. Is the background appropriate for the conceptional age and physiological state?
2. Look for left-right asymmetries in the background. Is one side suppressed in comparison to the other? Does one side have excessive delta activity in comparison to the other?
3. Look for sharp waves and spikes. Are they unifocal or multifocal? Unilateral or bihemispheric? Are they in the frontal or temporal region? Are they single or repetitive?
4. Look for possible epileptiform activity. Are there episodic suppressions due to desynchronization? Is there a stereotypic rhythm? Monomorphic alpha in neonates is usually a subcortically generated seizure discharge.
5. Look for changes in background with changes in state. An invariant pattern may be abnormal.
6. Can a possible abnormality be explained by a normal rhythm?

Normal Neonatal Electroencephalography

Wake and Sleep Cycle in Neonates

Normal term patterns of EEG activity are seen by 38-weeks conceptional age. At term, two stages of sleep are identified: quiet sleep (QS) and active sleep (AS). Quiet sleep is characterized clinically by absence of movement and regular respiration. Active sleep is characterized by small eye and body movements and less regular respirations. Active sleep is the equivalent of rapid-eye-movement (REM) sleep and QS is considered the equivalent of non-REM sleep.

Two EEG patterns are associated with QS. One is slow-wave sleep, in which continuous delta activity predominates, and the other is tracé alternant (TA), in which there are alternating periods of relative quiescence and bursts of sharply contoured theta activity. The bursts may be 3 to 6 seconds long. The interburst activity ranges from 5 seconds to almost 15 seconds. The TA pattern must be distinguished from a pathological burst suppression, or the normal discontinuous pattern of premature infants. The EEG in AS is characterized by theta activity with some delta and beta activity superimposed. During the course of a long sleep, the first AS period is higher amplitude than subsequent AS periods. The later AS periods have more theta and less delta.

Maturation of the Electroencephalography

The preceding characteristics of EEG are only true for term infants. The EEG background matures quickly from 29 weeks to 38 weeks. In general, the background becomes more continuous and wake-sleep states become distinct as the brain becomes more mature.

Twenty-two to Twenty-nine Weeks Conceptional Age

The EEG shows long periods of low-voltage activity punctuated by short bursts of higher voltage activity. The bursts are composed of mixed frequencies. Sharply contoured theta and faster frequencies can give the normal bursts an epileptiform appearance but it is normal. The interburst intervals may last up to two minutes, although intervals of less than one minute are more typical. When the bursts first develop, there is poor synchrony between the hemispheres. With full development, there is good interhemispheric synchrony.

The alternating bursts and low-voltage activity are termed *discontinuous*, and the pattern called *tracé discontinu* (TD). This pattern appears similar to the burst suppression pattern seen in some older patients with encephalopathy. The two are differentiated by knowledge of the conceptional age.

Twenty-nine to Thirty-one Weeks Conceptional Age

The interburst intervals of the TD pattern are now shorter in duration and less regular. The interburst periods have a higher amplitude than in younger premature infants. Sleep stages are more differentiated than in younger neonates, and TD is seen prominently in QS.

Delta brushes are prominent at this age. These are composed of a slow component in the delta range with superimposed fast rhythmic activity in the alpha or beta range. Delta brushes are most prominent in central and occipital regions, and are seen best in AS. Delta brushes resemble sleep spindles but are physiologically different. Sleep spindles are not prominent in REM sleep and are minimal in the occipital regions. Also, the disappearance of delta brush and subsequent development of frontal spindles argues against a common physiological substrate.

Thirty-two to Thirty-four Weeks Conceptional Age

The EEG during QS is still discontinuous, although the intervals of quiescence are shorter and less pronounced. Delta brushes are still present, and the spindle component is of higher frequency. Slow waves in the delta range are seen in posterior leads. Active sleep is still discontinuous. Chin EMG is reduced during AS, but is not a reliable indicator of state.

Multifocal sharp transients appear at this stage, occurring in the wake and sleep states. They are differentiated from pathological spikes by their widespread distribution and lack of repetitive discharge.

Thirty-four to Thirty-seven Weeks Conceptional Age

Non-REM sleep (QS) is still discontinuous, but the interburst intervals are progressively shorter. The burst/interburst time ratios are 1:2 to 1:3. REM sleep (AS) is virtually continuous, with delta predominating posteriorly and theta and faster frequencies anteriorly. For the first time, EMG becomes a reliable indicator of state, with low amplitude in REM sleep.

Multifocal sharp transients are less prominent and are replaced by frontal sharp transients (encoches frontales). These are of higher voltage than multifocal sharp transients.

The EEG is more reactive to external stimuli than at earlier ages. Stimulation causes attenuation of the background and frequently is followed by a change in state.

Thirty-eight to Forty Weeks Conceptional Age

Term infants have good differentiation between REM sleep, non-REM sleep, and wakefulness. During non-REM sleep, the discontinuous pattern now has a burst-interburst ratio of about 1 to 1. This is the mature TA pattern (Figure 17.1). Non-REM sleep may be characterized by a continuous

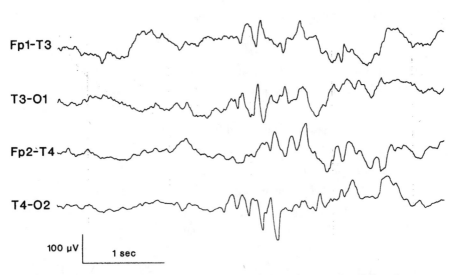

Fp1-T3

T3-O1

Fp2-T4

T4-O2

100 µV　1 sec

Figure 17.1 Tracé alternant pattern in a newborn. This pattern differs from premature patterns or burst suppression by the lack of profound suppression and the short interval between bursts.

Table 17.2   Lombroso's Classification of Abnormal Neonatal
Electroencephalogram Patterns

Abnormal EEG Patterns in Term Infants

I. Background abnormalities

    I-T-1   Inactive or isoelectric pattern

    I-T-2   Paroxysmal or burst-suppression pattern

    I-T-3   Low-voltage pattern through all states

    I-T-4   Interhemispheric amplitude assymetry

    I-T-5   Positive sharp waves

    I-T-6   Diffuse delta pattern

II. Ictal abnormalities

    II-T-1   Focal or unifocal ictal patterns

    II-T-2   Focal pseudo-beta-alpha-theta-delta ictal patterns

    II-T-3   Multifocal ictal pattern with abnormal background

    II-T-4   Low-frequency discharge pattern on low-amplitude background

    II-T-5   Lack of EEG discharges during clinical seizures

III. Abnormalities of states or maturation

    III-1   No recognizable states

    III-2   Changes in percentage of time of sleep state

    III-3   Abnormal maturation of sleep cycles and EEG

    III-4   Patterns of dysmaturity

Abnormal EEG Patterns in Preterm Infants

I. Abnormalities of background in preterm newborns

    I-P-1   Inactive or isoelectric pattern

    I-P-2   Paroxysmal or burst-suppression pattern

    I-P-3   Low-voltage pattern through all states

    I-P-4   Interhemispheric amplitude assymetry

    I-P-5   Positive sharp waves

II. Ictal EEG abnormalities in prematures

    II-P-1   Focal ictal patterns

    II-P-2   Focal pseudo-beta-alpha-theta-delta ictal patterns

    II-P-3   Multifocal ictal pattern

    II-P-4   Low-frequency ictal pattern

T = Term; P = Preterm.

Source: Lombroso 1987:725.

slow wave pattern rather than TA. This pattern is occasionally misinterpreted as encephalopathy in neonatal EEG.

Frontal sharp transients are less prominent, but may be seen until 2 months of age. Delta brushes are absent.

Abnormal Neonatal Electroencephalographic Patterns

Abnormal neonatal EEG patterns can be classified into abnormalities of maturation, epileptiform activity, and background abnormalities. Lombroso's classification based on these three categories is shown in Table 17.2. This combined numeric and alphabetic scheme can be used but does not substitute for a narrative impression.

Abnormalities of EEG Maturation

Dysmature means that the EEG patterns are not appropriate for the conceptional age. For example, a discontinuous pattern with an interburst interval of one minute is normal in a 29-week conceptional age (CA) neonate. However, this same pattern would be indicative of encephalopathy in a term infant. Persistent dysmaturity is associated with a poor neurologic outcome. Transient dysmaturity may be due to nonneurologic causes, and is not necessarily associated with brain damage.

Visual analysis of neonatal EEG allows for detection of only great discrepancies in EEG maturity. Quantitative analysis can detect more subtle dysmaturity; however, this is seldom necessary.

Abnormalities of state are difficult to diagnose in routine neonatal EEG. An invariant pattern is abnormal, but state change may not necessarily be captured during a twenty-minute routine EEG.

Epileptiform Activity in Neonates

Epileptiform activity may be focal, multifocal, or rarely generalized. Immaturity in cerebral myelination usually does not allow for generalization of epileptiform activity.

Focal discharges occur usually in central region, more often on the right than on the left. The discharges may occur singly or in trains at 5 to 10 per second. Focal epileptiform activity is differentiated from normal frontal sharp transients and multifocal sharp transients by consistent lateralization. Also, normal sharp transients never occur in trains. The focal discharges occasionally have a smooth contour and could be confused with an alpha or theta rhythm. However, sustained rhythmic activity is never normal in neonates of any conceptional age. The rhythm must be differentiated from the fast component of delta brushes by the absence of an underlying slow wave and duration of the discharge.

Focal discharges are usually associated with focal clonic seizures. The location of the focus may not necessarily correlate well with the clinical seizure activity. The prognosis for favorable neurologic outcome is good, since focal discharges in neonates do not necessarily indicate a structural lesion.

Most focal sharp waves are surface negative. Surface-positive waves are seen in some neonates with intracerebral hemorrhage. If the sharp wave is followed by a slow wave, the hemorrhage is most likely subarachnoid. If the sharp wave is not followed by a slow component, the hemorrhage may still be subarachnoid, but is more likely intraventricular, subependymal, or intraparenchymal.

Multifocal discharges are usually associated with an abnormal background, characterized by disorganization or suppression. The spikes can be single or multiple, occurring in trains similar to those of unifocal discharges.

The prognosis for good neurologic outcome is poorer for multifocal discharges than unifocal discharges. Seizures are usually clonic and may be subtle.

The chief differential diagnosis for multifocal discharges is normal multifocal sharp transients. The abnormal background is key to differentiation between these patterns.

Pseudo-beta-alpha-theta-delta is a descriptive term for a discharge that begins at 8 to 12/sec and gradually slows to 0.5 to 3/sec. The discharge may have a sharp appearance, but alternatively may have a smooth contour. This is an ictal pattern, with typical seizures being tonic, myoclonic, or subtle. The pseudo-beta-alpha-theta-delta rhythm usually indicates a poor prognosis and is commonly seen in patients with perinatal asphyxia.

Rarely, neonates may manifest seizures without any perceptible alteration in the background. The generator of epileptiform is probably subcortical, and the discharges are not projected to the surface. These infants usually have severe brain damage, explaining the lack of rostral projection of the activity.

Background Abnormalities in Neonates

Background abnormalities include excessive slow activity, low voltage, isoelectric recording, burst suppression pattern, and asymmetries. Excessive slow activity is difficult to discern, since neonates have prominent delta activity already. However, some infants with brain damage may have widespread delta. The slow background is present in wake and sleep states and reacts poorly to exogenous stimuli. This pattern is differentiated from normal delta activity by its widespread distribution and lack of reactivity. Normal delta is prominent anteriorly and is attenuated by exogenous stimuli.

Amplitude asymmetries are only significant if they approach 50% or more. The asymmetry usually indicates focal cerebral damage in the region of suppressed voltage. A common pitfall is misinterpretation of asymmetries due to extracranial hematomas or fluid collections. Subdural hematomas may suppress activity from one or both sides.

The isoelectric EEG is a confirmatory test for cerebral death. Guidelines for determination of cerebral death are presented in chapter 16, "Cerebral Death Studies."

The low-voltage record is unusual in neonates and suggests abnormalities in generation of electrical activity in the cortex. The technician needs to ensure that non-REM sleep is recorded, since normal REM sleep has a low-voltage background. Bilateral subdural hematomas may also produce bilateral attenuation of the background.

18 Troubleshooting in Electroencephalography

The most common difficulties encountered in routine electroencephalography (EEG) are related to noise, as when electrical activity of noncerebral origin contaminates the record. Other causes of poor EEG recordings are improper configuration of the EEG machine, improper electrode position, and unequal electrode impedances.

Noise

The most common sources of noise are muscle electrical activity, movement artifact, electrode pops, and 60-cycle interference. These will be considered individually.

Electrode Pops

Electrode pops are caused by a periodic discharge of a junction potential, either at the electrode-gel interface, or at the junction of dissimilar metals. The electrode, lead wire, and plug-in terminal are not necessarily of the same composition. When the junction potential suddenly discharges, current flows into the amplifier, producing a large fluctuation in recorded voltage. Current flow quickly stops since the discharge destroys the potential. This brief surge of current produces the "pop." Hair pins may cause electrode pops by the same mechanism.

Electrode pops are promoted by high electrode impedance, poor skin preparation, damaged electrodes or leads, contact with other metallic objects, and head movement.

60-Hertz Interference

Line voltage causes 60-Hz interference. Stray inductance and stray capacitance are described above, and in part I, "Basic Electronics." The differential amplifier rejects most of the 60-Hz interference; however, this rejection can be degraded by unequal electrode impedance.

In the hospital or office EEG laboratory, 60-Hz interference is minimized by careful selection of equipment location, grounding, and room shielding, if necessary. Therefore, use of the 60-Hz filter should not be needed. Portable studies in the intensive care unit may have significant contamination of the record by 60-Hz interference because of ventilators, intravenous (IV) infusion pumps, air beds, heating/cooling blankets, and monitoring equipment. To minimize these sources of noise, the following procedures may be helpful:

1. Unplug IV pumps. Most have battery backup for at least one hour. While on battery power, the direct current (DC) power supply will not interfere with the EEG in the same manner as the alternating current (AC) line power. Most modern pumps fill a reservoir periodically, and then slowly empty the reservoir into the patient. Most of the artifact arises during the brief filling period. This will not be interpreted as cerebral activity if the technician notes pump activity on the record.

2. Disconnect electrocardiogram (EKG) monitor. The EKG monitor not only adds noise by virtue of its line voltage, but its patient ground also prevents the EEG technician from placing a patient ground that is connected to the EEG machine. This would create a ground-loop, with potential for injury to the patient. If cardiac monitoring is essential, one channel of the EEG can be dedicated to EKG.

3. Heating/cooling blankets can virtually always be disconnected for the duration of the study. The recirculating water blankets produce much less artifact than the electric blankets or radiant heaters.

4. Ventilator artifact is uncommon, but movement artifact from chest-wall motion is not. If regular slow activity is seen in the EEG, activity from a chest-wall expansion sensor should be recorded for at least part of the study. Technicians will occasionally mark the record by hand, drawing an X with each respiration. While this may be helpful, there is a potential for error.

5. Air beds are a relatively new cause of noise (see Figure 12-8). The line power can cause 60-Hz interference, but more commonly, the blower motor creates a high-frequency artifact that can occasionally obscure the record. In most beds, the blower cannot be stopped without deflation of the mattress. While some beds have battery backup, this does not solve the high-frequency interference. If absolutely necessary, the bed can usually be deflated for the duration of the recording with no adverse effects on the patient. In our practice, this has seldom been necessary.

Before performing any of these maneuvers, the technician must check with the physician or nurse directly responsible for the patient's care.

Electrode Position

For routine EEG, twenty-three leads are placed on the head. Great potential for error exists in placement of the leads, especially if the technician does not measure the head. Also, there are only a limited number of lead colors, so switched leads can easily occur. Often, there is no obvious clue to misplaced electrodes. Error should be suspected if a field distribution does not make sense. Examples include a spike with no clear dipole distribution, a slow wave that reverses inappropriately, or alpha activity seen anteriorly which can be attributed to only one electrode. In this latter case, the interpreter must be sure that there is no skull defect in the region of a properly placed electrode, which could also give this anomaly.

Misplaced electrodes are common in institutions where leads are placed by technicians not well trained in EEG. For example, in our practice of telephone-transmission EEG recordings, we have seen a record where a well-modulated alpha was seen in anterior channels, and apparent eye-movement artifact posteriorly. The technician in the outside hospital had placed an electrode cap backwards on the patient's head.

Electrical Safety

General principles of electrical safety were discussed in detail in part I, "Basic Electronics." A few issues are specifically germane to electroencephalography. Of all EEG procedures, portable recordings in the intensive care unit pose the greatest risk to the patient. Leak current can flow from the EEG machine through the patient into other electrodes and grounds. The danger is greatest if the patient has a temporary pacemaker, where an externally grounded device has a lead within the heart. Electrocardiogram grounds are the most common route for flow of leak current. If a patient already has a ground, the ground electrode on the EEG machine should not be placed on the patient. This precludes testing of electrode impedance in most EEG machines and increases noise. However, acceptable recordings are usually possible. Alternatively, the leads to the cardiac monitor can be temporarily disconnected and the EEG ground placed normally but, of course, this is done only with the permission of the treating physician. Cardiac monitoring can be performed during the recording by using a channel on the EEG machine. Alternatively, a small battery-powered cardiac monitor may be used, since this does not provide a route for exit of leak current.

Nerve-Conduction Studies and Electromyography

19 □ □ □
□ □ □
□ □ □

Basic Principles of Nerve-Conduction Studies and Electromyography

Neurophysiological evaluation of nerve and muscle consists of nerve-conduction studies (NCS) and electromyography (EMG). Nerve-conduction studies have several components: nerve-conduction velocity, F wave, H reflex, blink reflex, repetitive stimulation, paired stimulation, and sympathetic skin response. Electromyography (EMG) consists of routine EMG, single-fiber EMG, and fiber-density determination. These techniques are discussed after a presentation of basic principles.

Equipment Required for Nerve-Conduction Studies and Electromyography

Most laboratories use self-contained instruments for electrodiagnosis that include an amplifier, an oscilloscope display, gain and filter controls, and a stimulator. Electrodes are plugged into a box that transmits signals to a preamplifier that in turn transmits signals to the main unit by a shielded cable. The signal is amplified, filtered, and either displayed on the oscilloscope or printed on paper. The oscilloscope display is divided in both the horizontal and vertical axes. The horizontal axis (time) has ten divisions representing seconds per division (sec/div); the vertical axis (voltage) has eight or ten divisions representing volts per division (volts/div). Tables 19.1 and 19.2 show recommended stimulating and recording settings for routine NCS and EMG, respectively.

Machines

Several different kinds of machines are available for routine NCS and EMG. The relative merits of specific machines will not be discussed, but some general features are desirable:

Table 19.1   Stimulus and Recording Parameters for Nerve-Conduction Studies

Parameter	Motor NCV	Sensory NCV	F Wave	H Reflex
Gain	2 mV/div	20 µV/div	200 µV/div	200 µV/div
Time base	2 ms/div	1 ms/div	10 ms/div	10 ms/div
LFF	10 Hz	10 Hz	10 Hz	10 Hz
HFF	32 kHz	2 kHz	32 kHz	32 kHz
Stimulus duration	0.2 ms	0.1 ms	0.2 ms	0.2 ms

NCV = Nerve-conduction velocity; LFF = Low-frequency filter; HFF = High-frequency filter.

Note: Available gain and filter settings differ between machines. Not all are able to provide the 32-kHz HFF setting. Lower setting is acceptable for most studies, although the waveform may be altered significantly. The main effect of a lower HFF setting is on amplitude. Minimal latency is virtually unaffected. The HFF settings for the F wave and H reflex are not as critical as for motor and sensory waves.

Table 19.2   Stimulus and Recording Parameters for Electromyography

Parameter	Resting	Motor Unit	Recruitment	Single Fiber
Gain	50 µV/div	200 µV/div	1mV/div	0.2–1 mV/div
Time base	10 ms/div	10 ms/div	10 ms/div	0.5–1 ms/div
LFF	10 Hz	10 Hz	10 Hz	500 Hz
HFF	32 kHz	32 kHz	32 kHz	32 kHz

LFF = Low-frequency filter; HFF = High-frequency filter.

Note: The HFF setting can be as low as 10 kHz for single-fiber EMG. An HFF of 20 kHz is acceptable for resting, motor unit, and recruitment recordings.

- Analog display
- Storage display
- Averaging
- Paper printout
- Repetitive stimulation
- Paired stimuli.

The method of display depends, to some extent, on personal preference. However, most clinical neurophysiologists prefer an analog display for EMG. Machines that use a digital display often have an annoying flicker. The storage display is usually digital. The machine should be able to display at least two stored traces on the screen in order to compare the responses to proximal and distal stimulation.

Averaging is helpful for sensory-conduction studies. The sensory nerve action potential is occasionally of low amplitude, and baseline noise can cause difficulty in the determination of latency. Averaging provides a smooth wave-form that is easier to interpret.

Paper printout is needed for the storage of waveforms if the machine lacks digital storage. Printouts of traces are especially important for repetitive stimu-lation, single-fiber EMG, and diagnosis of conduction block.

The machine should be able to deliver repetitive stimuli and paired stimuli. These are helpful for the diagnosis of disorders of neuromuscular transmission.

Machines for clinical neurophysiology are made by several vendors. The fea-tures and specifications are frequently changed, making any discussion almost instantly obsolete. Much of the difference between machines is in the ease of use. Be certain to perform studies on several machines before purchasing one.

Electrodes

Surface electrodes are used for routine NCS. The electrodes are stainless-steel, silver, or (occasionally) gold disks soldered to multistranded conducting wire (see Figure 19.1). The impedance is very low and the charge movement small, so that the use of silver-silver chloride electrodes, as used in EEG, is not necessary. Electrode gel is needed to reduce impedance and pre-vent artifact, because skin surface is irregular and hair interferes with conduc-tion. The gel is a malleable extension of the electrode, allowing electrical continuity between the ionic milieu of the skin and the electrode. Gel is also needed to reduce the impedance of the stimulating electrodes. The stimulus voltage passing through a high impedance can create sufficient heat to cause local tissue injury.

Ring electrodes are tight coils of stainless steel used to record or to stimu-late sensory action potentials from fingers. The coil is coated with conducting gel, wrapped around the finger, and cinched with a rubber or plastic fastener.

Needle electrodes (described in more detail in chapter 21, "Electromyogra-phy") are needles that are insulated except at the tip. The needle electrodes are inserted into the muscle to directly record muscle fiber and motor unit activ-

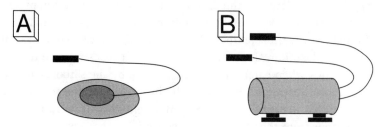

Figure 19.1 Electrodes. Diagrammatic representation of types of electrodes used in nerve conduction studies. *(A)* Disk electrode soldered to multistrand conduct-ing wire. *(B)* Bar electrode with two surface electrodes attached to the skin.

ity. Needle electrodes are usually reserved for EMG but may be helpful when recording from some nerves. Needle electrodes should not generally be used for stimulation because their high impedance can result in sufficient heat to damage tissue.

Surface electrodes are used in EMG for a ground and for reference to a monopolar needle electrode. Surface references are not needed in coaxial electrodes, because the reference is the barrel of the needle.

Principles of Nerve and Muscle Physiology

The theory needed to explain the generation of EMG activity is simpler than that needed to explain the generation of EEG activity. The important components of the motor system are:

- Motoneuron with motor axon
- Muscle fibers (extrafusal)
- Muscle spindle, including intrafusal muscle fibers
- Sensory neurons and axons that convey information from mechanoreceptors in the muscle to the spinal cord
- Spinal cord and higher centers.

Normal Neuromuscular Function

Motor Function
Input descending from the brain to the spinal cord activates the motoneurons. Action potentials that develop in the axon hillock of the motoneuron are transmitted to the nerve terminal by saltatory conduction. Calcium flows into the depolarized nerve terminal and promotes the release of acetylcholine (ACh) vesicles into the synaptic cleft. Acetylcholine binds to specific ACh receptors at the end-plate of the muscle fiber membrane and opens ionic channels that allow sodium and calcium into the cell and potassium and chloride out. The net effect of this ion flux is depolarization of the postsynaptic (muscle) membrane. Depolarization causes an action potential to be created in muscle fiber membrane adjacent to the end-plate that is propagated throughout the muscle fiber. The propagated potential releases calcium from the sarcoplasmic reticulum, which in turn causes muscle to contract. Contraction ends when calcium is taken back up by the sarcoplasmic reticulum. Activation of one motoneuron results in activation of every muscle fiber innervated by that neuron. The motor unit potential is the summation of the action potentials from the muscle fibers comprising that unit.

Most muscle fibers are extrafusal, outside of the muscle spindle. Some motoneurons activate intrafusal muscle fibers, whose contraction maintains the mechanoreceptor in a state of readiness to perform. The spindle ensures that extrafusal muscle fibers generate a desired level of force. If the force required to shorten a muscle is greater than expected, then contraction of the intrafusal muscle fibers stretches the muscle spindle, which sends signals to the spinal cord that promote further contraction of the extrafusal muscle fibers. This feedback loop assures that the muscle is appropriately shortened. The additional force is generated by recruitment of nonfunctioning motor units and increased rate of discharge of already functioning motor units.

Sensory Function

Nerve terminals are excited by the sensory stimulation and create afferent action potentials in sensory nerves. The impulses enter the dorsal horn where some information ascends the dorsal columns ipsilaterally, some ascends contralaterally, and some is used for segmental reflexes. Cell bodies of the afferent neurons are in the dorsal root ganglia.

Abnormal Neuromuscular Function

The possible sites of abnormal function of the peripheral nerves and muscle are:

- Motor and/or sensory neuron cell body
- Root
- Plexus and/or peripheral nerve axons
- Plexus and/or peripheral nerve myelin
- Neuromuscular junction
- Muscle.

Specific disorders characteristic of each lesion site are listed in Table 19.3. Degeneration of the cell body results in axonal degeneration and loss of innervation of the muscle fibers. With time, some muscle fibers are reinnervated by surviving motor axons. Others are not innervated, because of a limited ability of surviving axons to innervate extra muscle fibers. The membranes of actively denervated muscle fibers are unstable, causing the resting potential to fluctuate. These fluctuations occasionally result in spontaneous muscle fiber action potentials. Axonal degeneration causes the same physiologic changes in distal nerve and muscle as neuronal degeneration.

Lesions of myelin cause impaired saltatory conduction in peripheral nerves. Damaged myelin causes slowed conduction and, if severe, conduction block.

Muscle lesions cause instability of the muscle fiber membrane. The unstable membrane discharges spontaneously and may fail to activate from normal neuromuscular transmission. The tension generated by abnormal muscle fibers is reduced, so that more units must be recruited to generate the desired

Table 19.3   Sites of Damage in Nerve and Muscle

Site	Disorder
Neuron cell body	Amyotrophic lateral sclerosis
Root	Cervical or lumbar radiculopathy
Axonal neuropathy	Toxic neuropathy
Demyelinating neuropathy	Guillain-Barré syndrome
Neuromuscular junction	Myasthenia gravis
Muscle	Muscular dystrophy

force. This correction is partly conscious but largely automatic and is part of the feedback control mechanisms.

Basics of Nerve-Conduction Studies and Electromyography

Nerve-Conduction Studies

The time required for nerve conduction is measured by stimulation of a peripheral nerve and recording potentials from nerve or muscle. Details of methodology are presented in chapter 20. Normal values for nerve-conduction velocity (NCV) are established for all of the major nerves (see Table 19.4). An NCV is abnormal if it is more than 2.5 or 3 standard deviations from the mean.

Disorders of the myelin sheath slow the motor and sensory NCVs. Unraveling or fragmentation of the myelin reduces the impedance between spaces inside and outside the axon. This interferes with the electrotonic depolarization between nodes which is essential for saltatory conduction. Demyelinated axons do not have the capacity to conduct in the same way as unmyelinated fibers. Therefore, if severe enough, a demyelinating disorder can result in failure of transmission of impulses down the nerve.

Nerve-conduction velocities are typically normal or near normal in disorders of neuronal or axonal degeneration, because surviving axons conduct action potentials at a normal velocity. However, the amplitude of the compound action potential is often reduced, because the numbers of functioning axons is reduced. Disorders of muscle have normal NCS.

Electromyography

Electromyography is the recording of motor unit potentials (MUP). It can distinguish active from chronic denervation and myopathic from denervating disorders, as well as distinguish among several different types of myopathic disorders.

Table 19.4   Normal Data for Nerve-Conduction Studies

Nerve	Distal latency	NCV	Amplitude
Motor Nerve-Conduction Studies			
Median	≤ 3.8 ms @ 7 cm	≥ 50 m/sec	≥ 5 mV
Ulnar, below elbow	≤ 3.1 ms @ 7 cm	≥ 50 m/sec	≥ 5 mV
Ulnar, across elbow	—	≥ 50 m/sec	≥ 5 mV
Radial	≤ 3.4 ms @ 6 cm	≥ 50 m/sec	≥ 5 mV
Peroneal	≤ 6.0 ms @ 8 cm	≥ 40 m/sec	≥ 2.5 mV
Tibial	≤ 5.0 ms @ 10 cm	≥ 40 m/sec	≥ 2.6 mV
Sensory Conduction Studies			
Median	≤ 3.5 ms @ 13 cm	≥ 55 m/sec	≥ 10 μV
Ulnar	≤ 3.2 ms @ 11 cm	≥ 54 m/sec	≥ 10 μV
Radial	≤ 2.8 ms @ 10 cm	—	≥ 18 μV
Sural	≤ 4.2 ms @ 14 cm	≥ 42 m/sec	≥ 4 μV

Note: Distal latency is in units or milliseconds at the specified distance between stimulating cathode and active recording electrode. Nerve-conduction velocities (NCV) are in meters per second. Amplitude is in millivolts or microvolts.

Ulnar conduction across the elbow is usually compared to distal conduction and conduction on the contralateral side. A difference of 10 m/sec or greater is significant.

The instability in muscle fiber membrane potential which characterizes neuropathies and myopathies may occasionally reach threshold, producing a single muscle fiber action potential. These spontaneous potentials never occur in normal muscle at rest, and are called *fibrillation potentials* and *positive sharp waves.* These spontaneous potentials may not develop for three to four weeks after a nerve injury.

Normal motor unit potentials are biphasic in appearance and less than 15 ms in duration. In neuropathic conditions, new nerve sprouts reinnervate denervated muscle fibers. However, these nerves do not conduct as efficiently as the original connections, so potentials from these muscle fibers lag behind the potentials from the native muscle fibers. Therefore, the MUP has a polyphasic appearance with prolonged duration. Myopathic conditions produce MUPs of reduced amplitude because damaged muscle fibers may not respond to neuromuscular transmission. The MUPs are polyphasic in appearance but normal in duration.

A maximal voluntary contraction normally activates so many motor units that individual units cannot be identified. In neuropathic conditions, the number of motor axons is reduced, so there are fewer active motor units, but each is firing faster than normal. Myopathic conditions do not cause a loss of motor units but more motor units must be recruited to produce or maintain a given tension than in normal muscle.

20

□ □ □
□ □ □
□ □ □

Nerve-Conduction Studies

Methods of Routine Nerve-Conduction Studies

The stimulus for nerve conduction is a square-wave pulse that varies in duration and amplitude. Duration is varied by a control on the instrument. The standard duration is 0.2 ms. Longer duration stimuli (for example, 0.5 ms) can produce sufficient current to activate the nerve several millimeters distal to the stimulating electrode, and should not be used unless there is insufficient nerve activation with maximal voltage, for example, patients who are obese or have limb edema. Even then, the results must be interpreted with caution.

Stimulus voltage is varied continuously and can be set by controls on the instrument or on the stimulator handset. The maximal voltage output varies between instruments, but is usually 250 V. A brief direct current (DC) pulse of 250 V is not normally injurious to skin or neural tissues.

Motor Nerve-Conduction Velocity

Figure 20.1 shows a diagram of the techniques to study motor nerve-conduction velocity (NCV). The active recording electrode (G1) is placed over the midbelly of the muscle and the reference (G2) is placed approximately 2 cm distal to G1. Nerve stimulation evokes a compound motor action potential (CMAP) from the muscle. This is the summed potentials of multiple muscle fibers. The CMAP is sometimes called the *M response* (M for muscle), but *CMAP* is the preferred term. If the active recording electrode is not correctly placed, the major negative deflection of the CMAP may have an initial positive component. Determination of latency is then difficult because there is no initial negative deflection.

The stimulating electrodes, usually on a wand with two rigid electrodes, are placed on the skin over the nerve being tested. Depolarization is greatest beneath the cathode, which is placed distally to the anode. The ground is at-

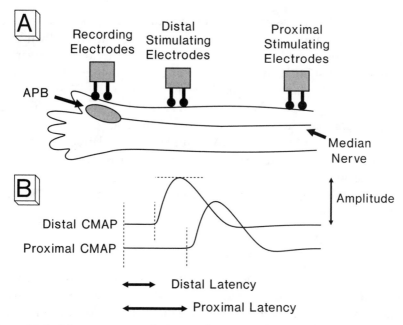

Figure 20.1 Motor nerve conduction velocity. *(A)* Recording is made from a muscle with the active electrode on the skin overlying the end-plate region. The nerve is stimulated at two locations, proximally and distally. The stimulator is oriented so that the cathode is closer to the muscle. *(B)* Simulated oscilloscope traces with proximal and distal stimulation. Dashed lines delineate the measurements made after data acquisition.

tached on the same limb. All electrodes are coated with electrode gel and fastened to the limb with tape or Velcro straps. The stimulating electrode is usually held in position by hand.

For motor NCV, the settings of the low-frequency filter is 10 Hz and the high-frequency filter is 32 kHz (see Table 19-1). The oscilloscope is set for 2 ms per horizontal division and 2 mV per vertical division.

After all electrodes are in place, the instrument is set to deliver repetitive stimuli at 1 Hz. The stimulus voltage is initially set to zero and then gradually increased. A CMAP gradually appears and grows larger in size and changes slightly in shape as the stimulating voltage increases. Eventually, further increases in voltage do not cause any change in CMAP amplitude. A stable response is assured if the voltage used is 25% greater than the voltage needed to produce the highest amplitude CMAP.

The following measurements are made of the CMAP:

- Latency from stimulation to takeoff of the CMAP
- Latency from stimulation to peak of the CMAP
- CMAP amplitude.

After these measurements are made, the stimulating electrode is moved to a more proximal location on the nerve. It is not necessary to gradually increase the voltage for this second round of stimulation. If the waveform is the same as with distal stimulation, then only one or two stimuli are needed. If the waveform is attenuated or has a different shape than the first CMAP, the examiner should increase the voltage to make sure that the changes are not due to incomplete activation. The same measurements are made on the CMAP with proximal stimulation as on the CMAP with distal stimulation. The distance between the two stimulating cathode positions is then measured along the course of the nerve.

When all of the measurements have been made, the motor NCV is calculated from the following formula:

$$NCV = \frac{Dist}{Pl - DL}$$

where PL is proximal stimulation latency, DL is distal stimulation latency, and Dist is distance between the stimulating cathodes. Latencies are measured in ms and distance in mm. Therefore, the final units of NCV are mm/ms, which is equivalent to meters/second (m/sec).

Sensory Nerve-Conduction Velocity

Sensory NCVs are measured more directly than motor NCVs (see Figure 20.2). Only one stimulating site is needed, because the delay caused by neuromuscular transmission and muscle contraction does not have to be subtracted. However, sensory NCVs require that either stimulating or recording electrodes be over a pure sensory portion of the nerve. Nerves that have pure sensory portions include the superficial peroneal, sural, and radial. Ring electrodes on the fingers are used for the median and ulnar nerves. Since there are no muscles in the fingers, recorded action potentials must be in cutaneous nerves.

Sensory NCVs can be performed with antidromic or orthodromic stimulation as long as they are done in a consistent fashion. Normative data is established for both directions of conduction. There is a slight discrepancy in the NCVs calculated with the two methods because of differences in the geometry of volume conduction. In general, orthodromic stimulation is recommended because there is less shock artifact and fewer nerve fibers are stimulated. Antidromic stimulation should be performed if no reproducible response is obtained from orthodromic stimulation.

The initial settings are stimulus frequency 1/sec, stimulus intensity zero, oscilloscope sweep speed 1 ms/div, and oscilloscope sensitivity 20 μV/div. The low-frequency filter is set at 10 Hz and the high-frequency filter at 2 kHz. The

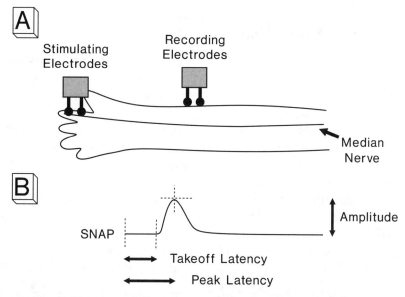

Figure 20.2   Sensory nerve conduction velocity. *(A)* Electrode placement. *(B)* Simulated oscilloscope traces of a sensory nerve action potential. Dashed lines delineate the measurements made after data acquisition.

stimulus voltage is gradually increased until a sensory neural action potential (SNAP) appears. When the potential no longer changes with increasing stimulus intensity, the trace is stored and the following measurements are made:

- Latency to takeoff of the potential
- Latency to peak potential
- Amplitude of the potential
- Distance between stimulating cathode and active recording electrode.

Sensory NCV is calculated by the following formula:

$$NCV = \frac{Dist}{LT}$$

where Dist is the distance between stimulating cathode and active recording electrode, and LT is the latency to takeoff of the potential. Unlike motor NCVs, both the takeoff and peak latencies of the SNAP can be used for interpretation. Takeoff latency more accurately represents conduction of the fastest fibers, so this is the preferred measurement. In our laboratory, we document both but predominantly use takeoff for interpretation.

Sensory NCVs may be normal in patients with very proximal lesions of nerve roots, especially avulsion, because the nerve fibers are damaged between the dorsal root ganglia and spinal cord. The connection between the ganglia and periphery is intact.

Effects of Age and Temperature on Nerve-Conduction Studies

The velocity of nerve conduction in the newborn is only half as fast as in adults. Velocity increases progressively and reaches adult speeds at approximately 3 years of age. After age 60, motor and sensory nerve-conduction velocities slow slightly.

Normative data are defined for normal temperature. Skin temperature of 34°C correlates with normal tissue and muscle temperature of 37°C. If the limb is cool, NCVs are slow. This is a common source of error when measuring NCV. There are two methods for dealing with the effect of temperature: (1) warm the extremity with an infrared lamp or forced air heater, or (2) correct the NCV for temperature. Add 5% to the conduction velocity for each degree below 34°C.

The second method is less desirable because of inherent errors in these calculations. The following guidelines should be followed when heating an extremity:

1. Do not heat too rapidly or the patient may suffer a skin burn.
2. Ensure that sufficient time has elapsed for warming before performing the study. The skin temperature can reach a desirable temperature before deeper structures are warmed. This is especially true in patients with peripheral vascular disease.
3. Turn the heat lamp off before performing the conduction study to eliminate artifact created by the lamp.

Interpretation of Abnormalities

Reduced Conduction Velocity

If either motor or sensory conduction velocity is slower than three standard deviations below the mean, the study is interpreted as abnormal. This indicates an abnormality in the myelin component of the nerve. Axonal neuropathies may cause mild slowing of nerve conduction, usually not more than 5 m/sec below the lower limit of normal.

Increased Distal Motor Latency

The motor distal latency is the time for conduction through the distal nerve plus neuromuscular transmission plus propagation of the muscle fiber action potential to the region under the recording electrode. Distal latency can be increased by demyelinating neuropathies, neuromuscular transmission defects, or dysfunction of the muscle fiber membrane. In practice, the most common cause for increased distal motor latency is demyelination or compression of the distal portion of the nerve.

Low-Amplitude Potentials

Low-amplitude CMAPs indicate a reduced number of functioning muscle fibers. This can be caused by motor units dropping out or by impaired excitation of muscle fibers. Decreased CMAP amplitude is seen in motor neuropathies, axonal degenerations, and myopathies.

Low-amplitude SNAPs indicate fewer functioning sensory axons. Sensory neural action potential amplitude is more variable than CMAP amplitude in normal people. Caution is needed when interpreting a sensory conduction study on the basis of amplitude alone. Lesions that significantly affect SNAP amplitude usually slow conduction as well.

Dispersed Waveform

A dispersed waveform is usually caused by a demyelinating process. Demyelination does not slow the conduction velocity of each axon uniformly. The result is a poorly synchronized nerve volley that accentuates the normal dispersion of the compound action potential. Axonal degeneration may also cause waveform dispersion when there is secondary demyelination.

Nerve-Conduction Velocities for Specific Nerves

Median Nerve

Median for motor NCV is calculated according to the formula cited previously. The active recording electrode (G1) is placed over the belly of the abductor pollicis brevis (see Figure 20.3). The reference (G2) is placed 2 cm distally. The cathode for distal stimulation is placed 7 cm proximal to G1 on the median nerve. The anode is placed 2 cm proximally. The cathode for proximal stimulation is placed over the median nerve proximal to the antecubital fossa. The anode is placed 2 cm proximal to this site. Normal distal latency is less than or equal to 3.8 ms. Normal motor NCV is greater than or equal to 50 m/sec.

Median sensory NCV is performed by using orthodromic stimulation. Stimuli are delivered to the fingers and recordings made from the median nerve at the wrist. Ring electrodes are placed on digits 2 or 3 for stimulation with the cathode as proximal as possible on the digit. The anode is 2 cm distal to the cathode. The active recording electrode (G1) is placed 13 cm proximal to the cathode and the reference (G2) is placed 2 cm proximal to the active electrode. The sensory NCV can also be measured by antidromic stimulation; however, the stimulus artifact is greater.

The median nerve is commonly studied for evaluation of suspected carpal tunnel syndrome. Absolute median motor distal latency and sensory NCV are usually abnormal. Some clinical neurophysiologists study incremental stimu-

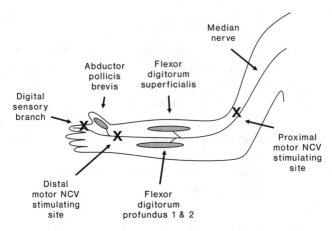

Figure 20.3 Median nerve anatomy. View of the medial aspect of the arm, showing innervation of the median-innervated muscles that are most important in neurophysiology. *X* marks refer to sites for stimulation, as labeled. Shaded areas represent approximate muscle positions. Sensory stimulation is delivered to the digital sensory branch.

lation across the carpal tunnel to document the lesion. Compound motor action potentials are recorded in response to stimulation at 1-cm increments, beginning at the site of distal stimulation for median motor NCV and progressively moving onto the palm. Each successive CMAP will have a little shorter distal latency. The latency disproportionately changing between two positions or a change in the waveform demonstrates evidence of median nerve compression in that segment. Normally, there is a latency change of 0.16 to 0.20 ms/ cm distance across the tunnel. However, abnormalities of incremental stimulation in the presence of normal distal latency are not convincing evidence of compression.

The main pitfall to median NCV studies is the Martin-Gruber anomaly. See chapter 27, "Troubleshooting," for a review of nerve anomalies.

Ulnar Nerve

For motor NCV, the ulnar CMAP is recorded from the abductor digiti minimi. G1 is placed over the belly of the abductor digiti minimi, approximately midway between the origin and insertion (see Figure 20.4). G2 is placed 2 cm distal to G1. Distal stimulation is on the ulnar aspect of the wrist, 7 cm proximal to G1. Proximal stimulation is delivered so that the cathode is just below the ulnar groove at the elbow. More proximal stimulation is delivered at least 10 cm proximal to the ulnar groove. Nerve-conduction velocities are calculated for the nerve segments between the wrist and groove, and across

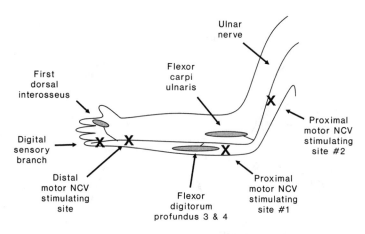

Figure 20.4 Ulnar nerve anatomy. Format is similar view to that of Figure 20.3.

the groove. A NCV across the elbow that is 10 m/sec less than that recorded distal to the elbow indicates an ulnar nerve lesion at the ulnar groove or cubital tunnel. If the NCV slows across the elbow, the contralateral side should be studied for comparison.

When measuring NCV across the elbow, a small error in measurement of distance or latency causes a large error in calculated NCV because of the short distance between stimulation sites. This error is exaggerated by the use of high-voltage, long-duration stimuli. High-voltage stimuli are volume-conducted through tissues and can depolarize the axonal membrane several millimeters from the cathode. Therefore, the distance measured on the skin may be longer than the distance between the site of activation and recording electrode. It is important to measure the distance with the elbow in the same position as it was during stimulation, usually flexed to 90 degrees.

Ulnar sensory NCV studies are performed by stimulating digit 5 (the little finger) using ring electrodes and recording from the ulnar nerve just above the wrist. Electrodes are placed as described for the median nerve, except that the distance between stimulating cathode and G1 is 11 cm. Antidromic stimulation can be performed if orthodromic stimulation fails to produce a measurable response or if this is the preference of the clinician.

Radial Nerve

Motor NCV is measured by recording from the extensor indicis. G1 is placed over the belly of the muscle. G2 is placed 2 cm distally. Needle electrodes can be used but are seldom required. The distal stimulation site is in the forearm, between the extensor carpi ulnaris and extensor digiti minimi, 10

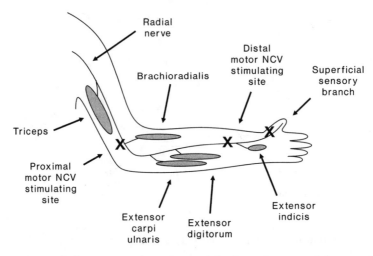

Figure 20.5   Radial nerve anatomy. View of the lateral aspect of the arm. Format is similar to that shown in Figure 20.3.

cm proximal to the styloid process. Proximal stimulation is just proximal to the antecubital fossa, between the biceps tendon and brachioradialis. Sensory NCV is measured by recording from the superficial sensory branch on the dorsum of the hand after stimulating from a more proximal site (see Figure 20.5).

Peroneal Nerve

The common peroneal nerve separates into superficial and deep peroneal branches. The superficial peroneal nerve innervates the peroneus longus and brevis, and terminates in sensory branches that supply the lateral aspect of the lower leg and the dorsum of the foot and toes.

The deep peroneal nerve, also called the anterior tibial nerve, innervates the tibialis anterior, extensor digitorum longus, extensor hallucis longus, peroneus tertius, and extensor digitorum brevis. The terminal sensory branches supply the skin over the first two toes. The extensor digitorum brevis is occasionally innervated by the accessory peroneal nerve, a branch of the superficial peroneal nerve.

Peroneal motor NCV is usually determined by recording from the extensor digitorum brevis (see Figure 20.6). Distal stimulation is in the lower leg, adjacent to the tendon of the tibialis anterior. Proximal stimulation is at the fibular neck. When the nerve is believed to be injured across the fibular neck, more proximal stimulation is then performed in the popliteal fossa. The NCV across the fibular neck is compared to the NCV distal to the neck. A difference of 10 m/sec or greater is abnormal.

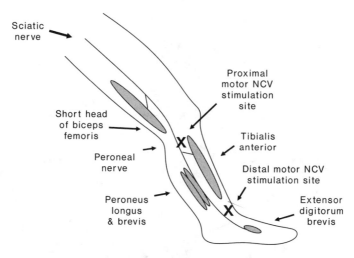

Figure 20.6 Peroneal nerve anatomy. View of the lateral aspect of the leg. Format is similar to that of Figure 20.3. The biceps femoris is not innervated by the peroneal nerve, strictly, however, this muscle is most important for evaluation of peroneal nerve function (see text).

Tibial Nerve

The tibial nerve innervates the medial and lateral gastrocnemius and soleus muscles and supplies sensation to those portions of the sole and dorso-lateral foot that are not served by the sural and superficial peroneal nerves. The tibial nerve also innervates most of the intrinsic muscles of the foot via the medial and lateral planter nerves. Tibial sensory NCVs are rarely performed and will not be discussed. Motor NCVs are performed by recording from the belly of the abductor hallucis muscle on the medial aspect of the foot (see Figure 20.7). Distal stimulation is delivered to the nerve as it passes behind the medial epicondyle, and proximal stimulation is delivered in the popliteal fossa.

Sural Nerve

The sural nerve is the only purely sensory nerve in the leg that is tested routinely. The sural is formed in the midcalf by the joining of branches from both the peroneal and tibial nerves. Sural sensory conduction is recorded from the nerve behind and slightly inferior to the lateral epicondyle. The stimulation site is on the posterior surface of the leg, 14 cm proximal to the recording site. There are no definite landmarks for the site of proximal stimulation, so some hunting may be needed. For most other NCV studies, the ground is placed proximal to the stimulating electrodes to minimize the potential for current to pass through the body. However, for sural sensory

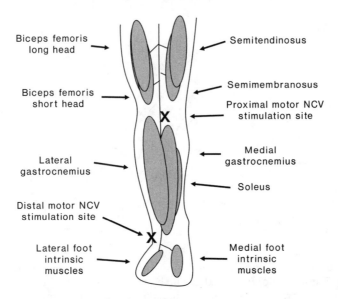

Figure 20.7   Tibial nerve anatomy. View of the posterior aspect of the left leg; therefore, left side is lateral and right is medial. Format is similar to Figure 20.3. The terminal motor branches of the tibial nerve are the medial and lateral plantar nerves, respectively.

NCV, the ground is frequently placed between the stimulating and recording electrodes. This minimizes the stimulus artifact (sometimes called "shock artifact"), which can obscure the sural SNAP.

F-Wave Study

The F-wave study tests conduction of motor axons proximal to the stimulation site. When motor nerves are stimulated for routine NCV studies, the stimulation creates action potentials that travel not only orthodromically toward the muscle, but also antidromically toward the motoneuron. The antidromic potential reaches the soma and depolarizes the dendrites. Depolarization is then conducted electrotonically back to the axon hillock, which is now repolarized. A new action potential is created and transmitted back to the muscle. The action potential activates the motor end-plate, causing action potentials in muscle fibers. This late response is the F wave (see Figure 20.8).

The recording electrodes for the F-wave study are placed in the same locations as for the motor NCV study. The stimulating electrode is over the nerve either proximally or distally. However, the stimulating electrodes are turned around, so that the cathode (negative pole) is toward the spine.

Normal values for F-wave conduction study are presented in Table 20.1.

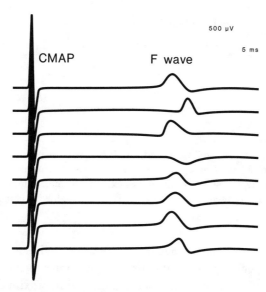

Figure 20.8 F-wave study of the median nerve. Stimuli are delivered to the distal median nerve. Recording is made from the abductor pollicis brevis. The responses to eight consecutive stimuli are shown in cascade format.

Interpretation is based on F-wave latency and the presence or absence of a response. Amplitudes are too variable to be of clinical use. Abnormalities of proximal conduction are unlikely to reduce amplitude without prolonging latency. Demyelinating peripheral neuropathies slow the F-wave response, since disorders that slow distal conduction also slow proximal conduction. An abnormal F-wave response is often the earliest electrophysiological measure in Guillain-Barré syndrome.

The F wave and CMAP can be used to calculate a proximal motor conduction velocity. The F-wave latency is the sum of the time for conduction to the spinal cord and back down to the muscle. If the CMAP is recorded from the same stimulating electrode position, this latency can be subtracted from the F-wave latency to derive the time from conduction to the cord and then back to the stimulating electrode. Therefore, proximal NCV can be calculated according to the following formula:

$$NCV = \frac{2 * Dist}{F - M}$$

where Dist is the distance from stimulating electrode to spine, F is F-wave latency, and M is the CMAP latency. Dist is needed only for the calculation of proximal NCV. However, even if proximal conduction is not calculated, patient height should be measured since F-wave latency varies with limb and spine length.

Table 20.1   Normal Data for F-Wave Studies

Nerve	Maximum Latency
Median	31 ms
Ulnar	31
Peroneal	51
Tibial	55

Note: During performance of the F-wave study, multiple trials are performed to a maximum of ten, or until one trial has a latency in the normal range. After ten trials, the shortest latency is reported on the data sheet. If this latency exceeds the maximum latency listed on the table, the study is interpreted as abnormal. This indicates slowing of proximal conduction in motor axons.

Several disorders increase F-wave latency. F-wave studies are useful in most patients with suspected peripheral neuropathy in order to compare proximal and distal conduction, but they are especially useful in proximal neuropathies such as the Guillain-Barré syndrome and chronic inflammatory demyelinating polyradiculoneuropathy (CIDP). The F-wave latency is usually normal in patients with axonopathies, radiculopathies, and plexopathies. Severe axonopathies with secondary demyelination increase F-wave latency, but the delay is small as compared to the axonal changes seen on EMG. The F wave may be absent in demyelinating neuropathies, because the afferent and efferent compound action potentials are dispersed.

H-Reflex Study

The H reflex is the electrophysiological counterpart of the tendon reflex. When the muscle is stretched by tapping the tendon, muscle spindles are activated and transmit afferent impulses to the spinal cord. Part of the reflex is generated by monosynaptic connections in the spinal cord, but much of the reflex is generated by polysynaptic pathways at both segmental and suprasegmental levels.

The H reflex is usually elicited from foot plantar flexors by stimulation of the tibial nerve. The patient lies prone with knees bent slightly. This is best done by placing a pillow under the feet. The stimulating electrode is in the popliteal fossa. The recording electrodes are over the soleus or medial gastrocnemius.

The oscilloscope time base is set at 10 ms/div and approximately 200 µV/div. The stimulator is set for repetitive stimulation at 1/sec or 0.5/sec and the voltage is gradually increased until a response is obtained from the muscle (see Figure 20.9). The first visible response, at approximately 30 ms, is the H reflex. As the stimulus voltage is increased further, a potential is recorded whose latency is much earlier than the H reflex. This early potential is the CMAP. The

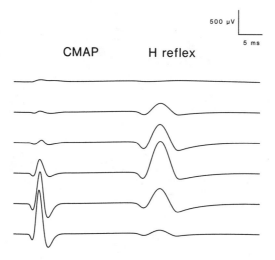

Figure 20.9 H-reflex study. Stimuli were delivered to the tibial nerve at the popliteal fossa and recordings made from the soleus. Each successive stimulus was of greater intensity. The first response is the H reflex because of the low threshold of afferent axons. At higher stimulus intensities, motor axons are directly stimulated, such that the CMAP predominates and the H reflex disappears.

H reflex disappears as the CMAP amplitude increases with increments of stimulus voltage.

Normal H-reflex latency is 35 ms or less, and interside differences should not exceed 1.4 ms. H-reflex amplitude varies greatly between patients and between sides and cannot be used for clinical interpretation. A delayed or absent H reflex is associated with both demyelinating and axonal neuropathies, and may also be seen as an isolated finding in patients with S1 radiculopathy.

The Blink Reflex

The blink reflex can be used to evaluate patients with lesions of the facial nerve, trigeminal nerve, or of the brainstem. However, neuroimaging is the preferred method to evaluate the brainstem, so the blink reflex is used predominantly to evaluate the cranial nerves.

Techniques of the Blink Reflex

Surface electrodes are placed in the following positions (see also Figure 20.10):

1. Active recording electrode (G1) is placed over the orbicularis oculi, usually below the eye.

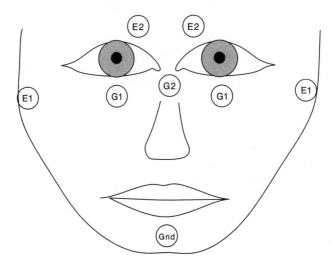

Figure 20.10   Blink reflex: electrode placement. G1 indicates the recording electrodes over the orbicularis oculi bilaterally. G2 is the reference for both
electrodes. E1 is the site for direct stimulation of the facial nerve, in front of the
ear. E2 is the site of stimulation of the supraorbital nerve.

2. Reference electrode (G2) is placed on the nose.
3. For direct response, stimulating electrodes are placed over the facial
   nerve anterior to the ear and slightly inferior to the external auditory
   canal, with the cathode distal.
4. For blink reflex, stimulating electrodes are placed over the supraorbital
   nerve with the cathode proximal.
5. Ground electrode are placed below the chin.
6. Electrodes are placed on the opposite side of the face corresponding to
   positions outlined in numbers 1 to 4, above.

Stimulating and recording parameters are detailed in Table 20.2. Stimulus
duration is 0.2 ms and intensity set high enough to establish a maximal direct
response. This direct response is the CMAP produced in the orbicularis oculi.

The Normal Blink Reflex

Before the blink reflex is performed, the facial nerve is stimulated
and the CMAP recorded from the orbicularis oculi. This is termed the *direct
response,* and is a test of the integrity of the efferent system. The usual latency
of the direct response is approximately 3 ms and should not exceed 4.1 ms.

Then, the supraorbital nerve is stimulated to evoke the blink reflex. Stimulation of the subraorbital nerve results in a response composed of two components:

Table 20.2 Blink Reflex: Stimulus and Recording Parameters

Parameter	Direct Response	Blink Reflex
Gain	1 mV/division	500 μV/division
Time base	1 ms/div	2 ms/div
Low-frequency filter	20 Hz	20 Hz
High-frequency filter	10 kHz	10 kHz
Stimulus duration	0.1 ms	0.1 ms

Note: Stimulus artifact may be further reduced by using an even shorter duration stimulus, for example, 0.05 ms, if your equipment allows this setting.

R1 and R2 (see Figure 20.11). R1 is a short loop reflex that is only projected ipsilateral to the stimulus. R2 is a longer loop reflex projected bilaterally.

Measurements are made of the latency of the direct response, R1, ipsilateral R2, and contralateral R2. R1 has a latency of about 10 ms and should not exceed 13.0 ms. R2 has a latency of about 30 ms and should not exceed 40 ms ipsilateral to the stimulus and 41 ms contralateral. Amplitudes are measured by some neurophysiologists; however, they are too variable to be used for clinical interpretation.

The blink reflex can be elicited not only by electrical stimulation but also by mechanical stimulation. A tap is delivered to the forehead by a hammer with a contact switch. The switch is connected to the EMG machine and triggers the sweep at the time of impact. The R1 with tap stimulation has an upper limit of normal of 16.7 ms. Mechanical stimulation usually offers no additional information over electrical stimulation, so this is not routinely performed.

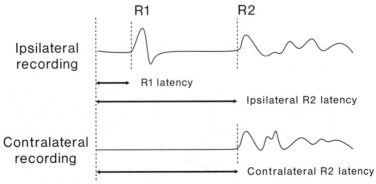

Figure 20.11 Blink reflex: normal response. R1 is seen only from the ipsilateral side. R2 is seen on both sides. The most important measurements are shown. Amplitude may be measured, but is not routinely used in analysis.

Interpretation of the Blink Reflex

Guides to the interpretation of the blink reflex are as follows:

1. Prolonged direct response with otherwise normal latencies indicate a lesion of the facial nerve, such as Bell's palsy.
2. Prolonged R1 indicates a lesion in the reflex pathway from trigeminal nerve to facial nerve. Facial nerve lesions also prolong R1, but are distinguished from brainstem or trigeminal nerve lesions because the direct response is prolonged as well. If the contralateral R2 is normal, then the afferent limb in the trigeminal nerve is normal, and a brainstem lesion is likely.
3. If the latency of the direct response is normal, but the latencies of R1, ipsilateral R2, and contralateral R2 are prolonged, a lesion of the trigeminal nerve is likely, but brainstem lesions cannot be excluded.

Sympathetic Skin Response

The sympathetic skin response is not strictly a nerve conduction. It is used to test the integrity of the sympathetic nervous system in patients with suspected autonomic neuropathy.

Electrodes are placed on the palm, not overlying any particular muscle. The leads are fed to a machine capable of recording DC potentials. Gain is set to approximately 20 μV/div with a sweep speed of 200 ms/div. The patient is asked to take a deep breath and then let it out. After a latency of a few seconds, there is a DC potential with the palm negative compared to the dorsum of the hand. The wave declines over about 5 seconds.

The study is interpreted as normal if the response is present, abnormal if the response is absent. No interpretation is made on the basis of amplitude or latency.

Guidelines for Efficient Nerve-Conduction Studies

Nerve-conduction studies must be individually designed to answer clinical questions. Recommended studies for specific, common neuromuscular disorders are presented in chapter 23, "Evaluation of Common Neuromuscular Problems." The following timesaving suggestions are applicable to virtually all conduction studies.

1. If you do not know the patient prior to the examination, take a brief history and do a directed neurologic examination. Time invested in clinical evaluation saves time by directing the electrical studies and maximizes the information derived.

2. Measure and mark the limbs for all anticipated nerve-conduction studies before starting.
3. Gradually increase the stimulus voltage during the initial study so that the patient is not surprised by the shock. Once the optimal voltage is established, use it immediately for subsequent nerve-conduction studies. There is no clinical value to "sneaking up" on the CMAP or SNAP.

Some neurophysiologists think that patients adjust to electrical stimuli over time. However, studies in animals and humans suggest that each successive electrical shock is progressively less well tolerated. The nervous system would rather have one adequate shock than many incremental stimuli.

21 ⬚⬚⬚ ⬚⬚⬚ ⬚⬚⬚

Electromyography

Technical Requirements

Electrodes

The three commonly used electromyographic (EMG) electrodes are monopolar, coaxial, and single fiber (see Figure 21.1). A monopolar electrode consists of a fine needle that is fully insulated with the exception of a very small region at the tip. The insulating material is usually a polymer plastic. The end of the wire opposite the needle point is soldered to multistranded wire that connects to the amplifier. The monopolar needle requires a reference, so a disk electrode is fixed on the skin overlying the study muscle, as described in chapter 20, "Nerve-Conduction Studies." A ground electrode is also placed on the skin proximal to the recording electrodes.

A coaxial electrode is composed of a fine wire inserted through the barrel of a hollow hypodermic needle. The wire is insulated, so that it does not touch the barrel of the needle. The recording surface is a small exposed portion of wire on the bevel of the needle, held in place by epoxy or a similar cement. The opposite end of the wire is soldered to multistranded connector wire. The barrel of the needle is also soldered to another wire, so that the barrel can serve as reference for the active recording surface. A ground electrode, but not a surface reference, is needed.

A single-fiber electrode is composed of a hollow needle with one or more insulated wires inserted through the barrel. The wires are turned and exposed on the side of the needle. This gives greater stability in longer-term recordings than when the electrode surface is on the bevel. The barrel serves as the reference for the single-fiber electrode.

Electromyography Machine Settings

The low-frequency filter is typically set to 10 Hz and the high-frequency filter to 20 kHz. Most EMG instruments have a multiposition switch, so that high- and low-frequency filters are simultaneously selected. The oscilloscope is set for 10 ms/div; the ten horizontal divisions provide a total sweep

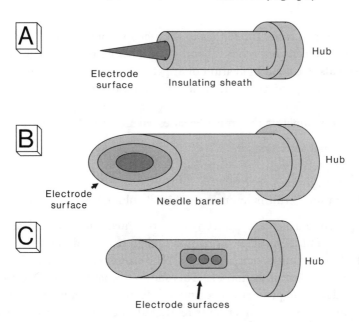

Figure 21.1   EMG electrodes. *(A)* Monopolar. *(B)* Coaxial. *(C)* Single fiber.

time of 100 ms. The sweep rate of 10/sec is selected because it is the fastest sweep that is still below the flicker-fusion-frequency of the human eye (about sixteen frames per second). This is necessary for accurate visual analysis of the EMG. At faster frequencies, the traces appear fused, making it impossible to tell whether two potentials are on the same or subsequent traces.

Gain is first set at 50 μV/div to inspect resting activity, because the amplitude of fibrillation potentials may be only 50 μV. Analysis of single motor units requires a gain of 200 μV –1 mV/div.

Electromyography Techniques

The EMG machine must be turned on before any electrodes are placed on the patient in order to avoid surges of current through the patient. The ground electrode is placed on the limb, proximal to the muscle to be studied. If a monopolar electrode is used, the reference is placed adjacent to the insertion point of the needle. Delagi et al. (1980) is an excellent reference to the landmarks for needle insertion in specific muscles. The needle is inserted through the skin and into the muscle before the electrode junction box is switched on. If the box is switched on before insertion, the open loop between active and reference electrodes creates high voltage artifact.

Electromyographic signals are usually analyzed by visual and auditory inspection. The clinical neurophysiologist watches as signals are displayed on the screen in real time, and listens to the signals from the audio monitor. Experienced clinicians often hear abnormalities before they are seen. The pitch of the signals is a good indication of "upstroke velocity," the rate of voltage change during a potential. It indicates the proximity of the electrode to the muscle fibers.

The four parameters that must be assessed are:

- Insertional activity
- Resting activity
- Single motor unit analysis
- Motor unit recruitment during maximal voluntary contraction.

The patient is asked to completely relax the muscle in order to assess resting activity. A minimal muscle contraction is then requested in order to evaluate individual motor unit potentials (MUPs). The examiner's hand should be placed to oppose the action of the muscle. This shows the patient how to contract the muscle and helps to prevent dislodging the electrode by limb movement. Next, a maximal voluntary contraction is requested to evaluate motor unit recruitment. The limb must be held firmly to minimize movement.

Normal Electromyographic Activity

Insertional Activity

Normal insertional activity consists of a brief discharge of multiple muscle fiber action potentials. The duration is usually less than 500 ms, with abrupt onset and termination. An example of normal insertional activity is illustrated in Figure 21.2.

Insertion may provoke potentials that look like fibrillation potentials and positive sharp waves. These are the potentials of single muscle fibers, and are not abnormal unless the discharge continues after needle movement has stopped.

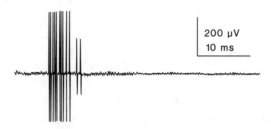

Figure 21.2 Normal insertional activity. The burst of activity was due to advancement of the needle electrode.

Spontaneous Activity

Normal muscles do not have spontaneous activity at rest. Persistent MUPs may occasionally be mistaken for abnormal spontaneous activity. Ensure that the patient has completely relaxed the muscle before interpreting abnormal spontaneous activity. Silencing of the muscle can occasionally be facilitated by contraction of an antagonist.

Motor Unit Potentials

The patient is asked to contract the muscle enough to activate a few motor units. Each discharge is a MUP. (Sample MUPs are shown in Figure 21.3.) The amplitude of the MUP depends on the number of muscle fibers innervated by the motor axon, and the proximity of the recording electrode to these muscle fibers. A typical MUP amplitude is 200 mV or greater. Amplitude is not as important as morphology in diagnosis. Most normal motor units are biphasic or triphasic. Up to 15% of motor units may be polyphasic before the muscle is classified as abnormal. The duration of most MUPs is usually less than 10 ms, and should not exceed 15 ms.

Recruitment Pattern

With increasing volitional muscle contraction, motor units discharge faster and more units are recruited. With maximal contraction, so many units are activated that the baseline is obliterated. This is called a *full interference pattern.*

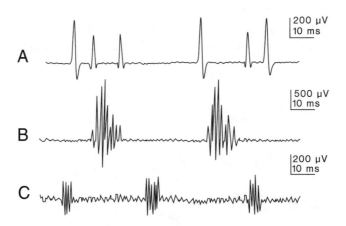

Figure 21.3 Motor unit potentials. Various examples of motor unit potentials. *(A)* Normal units. *(B)* Neuropathic units. *(C)* Myopathic units.

Abnormal Electromyographic Activity

Table 21.1 shows most of the common EMG findings, their origin, and their interpretation. Table 21.2 shows the expected EMG findings with neuropathic and myopathic disorders.

Abnormalities of Insertion

Increased Insertional Activity

Increased insertional activity indicates an exaggerated discharge, often with increased duration, such that the firing continues substantially after the end of electrode movement. None of the individual potentials is inherently abnormal; it is the repetitive and prolonged discharge that is abnormal.

Decreased Insertional Activity

Decreased insertional activity indicates a reduction in total activity with electrode movement, most common when there are few functioning muscle fibers, such as in long-standing denervation. An attack of periodic paralysis can result in abolition of insertional activity, since the muscle fibers are relatively inexcitable. Complete absence of insertional activity is more commonly caused by a faulty electrode than by absence of functioning muscle fibers.

Abnormal Spontaneous Activity

Fibrillation Potentials

Fibrillation potentials are single muscle fiber action potentials generated by abnormal spontaneous fluctuations in membrane potential that occasionally reach threshold (Figure 21.4). The potentials occur with a (more or less) random frequency, so that on the audio monitor they sound like rain drops. Fibrillation potentials occur at rest in patients with active denervation

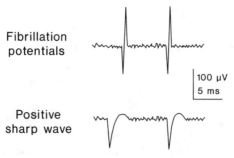

Figure 21.4 Abnormal spontaneous activity. Fibrillation potentials and positive sharp waves.

Table 21.1   Common Electromyographic Findings

Resting Activity	Origin	Interpretation
Fibrillation potential	Single muscle fiber action potential. Due to membrane potential instability.	Neuropathy or myopathy
Positive sharp wave	Single muscle fiber action potential	Neuropathy or myopathy. May appear sooner than fibrillations with denervation.
Fasciculation	Spontaneous discharge of a motor unit. Due to motoneuron or axon action potential.	Neuropathy or motor neuron disease. Normal in some individuals.
Myotonia	Repetitive discharge of muscle fibers	Myotonic dystrophy, myotonia congenita, and some with periodic paralysis
Complex repetitive discharge	Repetitive discharge of muscle fibers	Neuropathy or myopathy
Motor Unit Activity	*Origin*	*Interpretation*
Brief small-amplitude polyphasic motor unit potential	Reduced number of functioning muscle fibers and dispersal in time to activation	Myopathy
Long-duration polyphasic motor unit potential	Increased number of muscle fibers innervated by an axon with dispersed activation	Neuropathy. Chronic denervation with motor unit reorganization.
Maximal Contraction	*Origin*	*Interpretation*
Reduced recruitment	Reduced number of motor units	Neuropathy. Often is also rapid discharge of single motor units.
Early recruitment	Reduced tension output of each unit, requiring recruitment of more units and faster discharge	Myopathy

and with myopathies. Basic mechanisms of the membrane potential fluctuations were discussed in chapter 19, "Basic Principles of Nerve-Conduction Studies and Electromyography."

Fibrillation potentials are brief biphasic waves with an initial negative component followed by a positive component. Amplitude is 20 to 200 µV with a duration of 1 to 5 ms.

Table 21.2 Electromyogram Abnormalities

Abnormality	Fibs	Fascics	Polys	BSAPs
Acute denervation	+	−	−	−
Chronic denervation	±	±	+	−
Myopathy	+	−	−	+
Myotonia	−	−	−	−
NMJ transmission defect	±	−	−	±

Fibs = Fibrillation potentials and positive sharp waves; Fascics = Fasciculations; Polys = Long-duration polyphasic motor unit potentials; BSAPs = Brief small-amplitude polyphasic motor unit potentials; NMJ = Neuromuscular junction.

Fibrillation potentials occur at rest, but may not be present at all recording locations within a given muscle. Multiple places in each muscle must be examined. Fibrillation potentials may not appear for three to four weeks after a nerve injury.

Positive Sharp Waves

Positive sharp waves are single muscle fiber action potentials that look different than fibrillation potentials. Unlike fibrillation potentials, the initial deflection is positive, followed by a return to baseline. There may be a small negative wave after the positive component, but the positive deflection is predominant. The frequency is random, as are fibrillation potentials.

Positive sharp waves, like fibrillation potentials, are prominent in active denervation and in myopathies. The different appearance of the two waveforms may be explained by the location of the recording electrode. The fibrillation potential is biphasic because of the passing extracellular negativity created by propagation of the muscle fiber action potential. The membrane adjacent to the positive sharp waves may not be able to sustain an action potential, either due to focal damage from the underlying condition or to membrane deformation due to the electrode. Therefore, the action potential approaches the injured area but cannot excite it. The electrode sees the electrotonic potential that is trying to depolarize the membrane. This potential is an outward current, producing a positive extracellular field potential.

Fasciculations

Fasciculations are due to the spontaneous discharge of single motor units. The conformation of the MUP may be normal, or may have a neuropathic appearance. Fasciculations are differentiated from voluntary

MUPs by their pseudorandom frequency. The morphology and amplitude of fasciculation potentials may fluctuate, probably due to a shifting generator of the discharge.

Fasciculations are seen in normal individuals and in those with chronic denervation, most usually motor neuron disease. They should not be interpreted as abnormal without other EMG evidence of chronic denervation. Pathologic fasciculations often have a polyphasic appearance and discharge irregularly at an average interval of 3.5 seconds. Nonpathologic fasciculations discharge at a mean interval of 0.8 seconds.

Myokymia
Myokymia is an involuntary repetitive discharge of a single motor unit at a frequency of 30 to 40/sec. The muscle moves under the skin, giving a rippling or quivering appearance on examination.

Myokymia occurs in several denervating disorders, but is most common in the following conditions: multiple sclerosis, brainstem glioma, radiation plexopathy, Guillain-Barré syndrome, and gold neuropathy. The myokymia is localized to the face in multiple sclerosis and brainstem glioma. Myokymia occurs in radiation plexopathy but not in neoplastic infiltration of the brachial plexus, and its presence can be used as a distinguishing feature. Myokymia occasionally occurs in the eyelid of normal individuals.

Myotonic Discharges
Myotonic discharges are repetitive muscle fiber action potentials. Needle movement evokes the discharges, probably by membrane deformation and resultant depolarization (Figure 21.5). The frequency waxes and wanes, and has been described as having a "dive-bomber" sound on the audio monitor.

The repetitive discharge is probably due to an abnormality in chloride conductance. Chloride is localized predominantly in the extracellular space. At the end of an action potential, the membrane is repolarized by closure of sodium channels and opening of potassium channels. The potassium efflux is responsible for the transient hyperpolarization that follows an action poten-

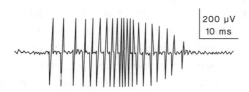

200 μV
10 ms

Figure 21.5 Myotonic discharges.

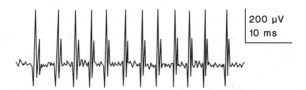

200 μV
10 ms

Figure 21.6 Complex repetitive discharges. Polyphasic potentials discharge repetitively. The frequency does not wax and wane as do myotonic discharges.

tial. As the potassium conductance falls to baseline, the membrane potential depolarizes toward normal. Normally, chloride conductance serves to keep the membrane from reaching threshold. If the chloride conductance is reduced, then the depolarization due to inactivation of potassium channels can result in another action potential. This cyclic depolarization, action potential, and repolarization occurs until the depolarization fails to reach threshold.

Myotonic discharges are seen in patients with myotonic dystrophy, myotonia congenita, paramyotonia congenita, and hyperkalemic periodic paralysis. Patients with inflammatory myopathies or acid maltase deficiency may have EMG evidence of myotonic discharges without clinical myotonia.

Complex Repetitive Discharges

Complex repetitive discharges are waxing and waning high-frequency synchronous discharges of several muscle fibers (Figure 21.6). Amplitudes range from 50 μV to 1 mV, and discharge rates from 5 to 100/sec. Total discharge duration may be a few seconds. Older terms, which should not be used, are *pseudomyotonia* and *bizarre high-frequency discharge*. Complex repetitive discharges are seen commonly in chronic denervation and in some patients with myopathies. They can rarely occur in otherwise normal individuals, and should not be interpreted as abnormal in the absence of other EMG abnormalities.

Abnormal Motor Unit Potentials

Neuropathic Motor Unit Potentials

Acute denervation, before reinnervation has occurred, results in loss of motor units. Surviving motor units have essentially normal function. Therefore, motor unit potential analysis is usually normal unless denervation is complete, and then there are no motor unit potentials.

Denervated muscle fibers are eventually reinnervated by sprouts of nearby surviving axons. Since the number of muscle fibers innervated by each surviving motor axon is increased, the amplitude of the reconstituted motor unit potential is often greater than normal. The new connections are often not activated synchronously with the original connections, so the MUP is usually polyphasic and of increased duration (Figure 21.3). High-amplitude, long-duration polyphasic is the hallmark of chronic denervation.

Myopathic Motor Unit Potentials

The instability of muscle fiber membrane potentials with myopathy results in alteration in conformation of the motor unit potentials. Some muscle fibers are irreversibly depolarized and fail to be activated by neuromuscular transmission. This failure results in motor unit potentials of low amplitude (Figure 21.3). In addition, the loss of some muscle fibers and the asynchronous activation of remaining damaged fibers results in polyphasic MUPs whose duration is not prolonged, as it is for neuropathic units. Myopathic MUPs are sometimes called *brief small-amplitude polyphasic potentials* (BSAPs or BSAPPs). While this term is discouraged by some neurophysiologists, it is a good descriptive term. Unfortunately, the association of BSAPs with myopathies is so strong in some minds that alternative interpretations are not considered. Similar MUPs can be seen in some patients with denervation, especially early, due to desynchronization of terminal nerve conduction.

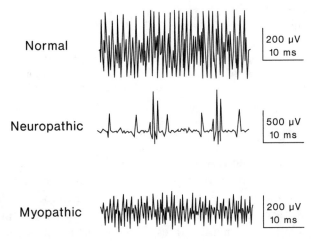

Figure 21.7   Recruitment patterns. Normal recruitment shows a mixture of motor unit potentials discharging at a high rate. Recruitment in neuropathic conditions is characterized by a reduced number of units. Units are polyphasic. Recruitment in myopathic disorders is characterized by low-amplitude potentials with a high frequency of discharge. A key is development of the full recruitment pattern with relatively weak contraction.

Table 21.3   Muscles Commonly Studied in Electromyography

Muscle	Nerve	Plexus	Root
Upper Extremity			
Abductor pollicis brevis	Median	MC	C8, T1
Biceps	Musculocutaneous	LC, UT	C5, C6
Deltoid	Axillary	PC, UT	C5, C6
Extensor digitorum communis	Radial	PC, MT, LT	C7, C8
First dorsal interosseus	Ulnar	MC, LT	C8, T1
Infraspinatus	Suprascapular	UT	C5, C6
Pronator teres	Median	LC, UT, MT	C6, C7
Serratus anterior	Long thoracic		C5, C6, C7
Supraspinatus	Suprascapular	UT	C5, C6
Triceps	Radial	PC, MT, LT	C7
Lower Extremity			
Extensor digitorum brevis	Peroneal	SP	L5-S1
Gluteus medius	Superior gluteal		L4-S1
Medial gastrocnemius	Tibial	SP	S1-2
Peroneus longus	Peroneal	SP	L5-S2
Rectus femoris	Femoral	LP	L2-4
Short head of biceps femoris	Peroneal	SP	S1-2
Tibialis anterior	Peroneal	SP	L4-5
Vastus medialis	Femoral	LP	L2-4

MC = Medial cord; LC = Lateral cord; PC = Posterior cord; UT = Upper trunk; MT = Middle trunk; LT = Lower trunk; SP = Sacral plexus; LP = Lumbar plexus.

Abnormal Recruitment

Reduced Recruitment

Reduced recruitment indicates a decrease in functioning units. Single units can be identified and these are often firing more rapidly to make up for the lack of recruitable units (Figure 21.7). Reduced recruitment is seen predominantly in axonal neuropathies but may also occur in demyelinating neuropathies if some motor axons fail to transmit.

Early Recruitment

Early recruitment means that many units are recruited at an abnormally low level of effort (Figure 21.7). This is typical of myopathies. The muscle contractions are ineffectual, so that additional units are recruited to generate the desired force. These units are often decreased in amplitude and produce an interference pattern that is reduced in amplitude but still able to obliterate the baseline.

Electromyographic Testing of Specific Muscles

The most commonly tested muscles are listed in Table 21.3. The selection of muscles for examination is based on the clinical question, and is discussed further in chapter 23, "Evaluation of Common Neuromuscular Problems."

22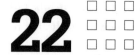

Special Tests of Neuromuscular Transmission

Repetitive Stimulation

Repetitive stimulation is a test of neuromuscular transmission and is indicated for patients with progressive weakness without sensory loss, patients with easy fatigability, and patients who have activity-dependent weakness.

Physiology

Normal neuromuscular transmission is one-to-one, that is, every motor axon action potential results in an action potential in each muscle fiber of the motor unit. This relationship fails at high rates of stimulation because some muscle fibers become refractory. The amplitude of the compound motor action potential (CMAP) then declines progressively, "the decremental response."

Normal individuals do not show a decremental response at stimulus rates less than 20/sec, but people with myasthenia gravis fail to fire repetitively even at low rates of stimulation. This is because there are an insufficient number of receptors available for binding with acetylcholine.

Unlike myasthenia gravis, botulism and the myasthenic syndrome are presynaptic defects in neuromuscular transmission caused by impaired mobilization or release of acetylcholine. The amount of transmitter released can be increased by repetitive stimulation at a fast rate, probably due to facilitated transmitter mobilization by the "priming" action potential.

Repetitive Stimulation at Slow Rates

Methods

Repetitive stimulation at slow rates is usually performed at 3/sec. Several different protocols have been suggested; I prefer the following:

1. Tape electrodes over the muscle under study with the active electrode (G1) on the belly, and the reference (G2) distal.
2. Deliver a train of nine or ten pulses at a rate of 3/sec. Photograph or print the display.
3. Maximally exercise the muscle for 1 minute.
4. Repeat the trains of repetitive stimuli at intervals of 1 minute until 5 minutes after the exercise.

Analysis of the responses can be performed in several ways. The most accurate is to determine the area under the curve of the CMAP, essentially integrating the potential. The CMAP is produced by a bipolar recording. The negative deflection indicates depolarization and the positive deflection indicates repolarization of the same muscle fibers. Therefore, only the negative portion of the CMAP is integrated. The negative area under the curve is thought to better correlate with the number of muscle fibers being activated than the measurements of the peak amplitudes. Most modern EMG machines perform this calculation automatically. The largest decrement is usually between the first and fourth or fifth responses.

The abductor digiti minimi, innervated by the ulnar nerve, is usually selected for repetitive stimulation studies, but the trapezius may be more sensitive to transmission defects. The spinal accessory nerve is stimulated at the base of the sternocleidomastoid muscle. G1 is placed on the belly of the upper portion of the trapezius, and G2 can be placed near the acromion. The patient exercises by holding onto the bottom of the chair with both hands and pulling the shoulders upward.

Interpretation

The repetitive stimulation study is considered abnormal if there is more than a 10% decrement from the first to fourth stimuli (see Figure 22.1). After the fifth stimulus, the CMAP amplitude may increase, with the responses to the ninth stimulus being near the level of the first.

Repetitive stimulation is used mainly for the diagnosis of myasthenia gravis. The decremental response is greater than 10%, but is not necessarily seen in all muscles. There are two reasons why spinal accessory nerve stimulation of the trapezius is more sensitive than ulnar nerve stimulation of the abductor digiti minimi: (1) distal muscles are less often affected than proximal muscles; and (2) distal muscles are more likely to be cool, and cooling of nerve and muscle can reduce the decrement to normal range.

Decremental responses occur in other disorders of neuromuscular transmission (partial denervation, myasthenic syndrome, botulism), and have been reported in multiple sclerosis. However, repetitive stimulation is not used for the diagnosis of multiple sclerosis.

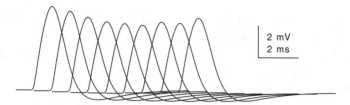

Figure 22.1 Repetitive stimulation at low rates. Responses to stimuli delivered at 3/sec are shown in overlapping format. This patient has a decay between responses 1 and 4.

Repetitive Stimulation at Fast Rates

Methods

Repetitive stimulation at fast rates is too painful to be used routinely in clinical testing. Its greatest use is in the diagnosis of botulism and myasthenic syndrome, although paired stimuli may provide similar information. Electrode placement is the same as described above for repetitive stimulation at slow rates. The stimulus rate is 20 to 30/sec, and the responses are recorded and analyzed for decrement or increment, as previously described.

Interpretation

Normal muscles show no significant increment or decrement in response to nerve stimulation at 20 to 30/sec. Faster frequencies are not used because a decremental response may appear when muscle fibers are no longer able to keep up with the rate of nerve activation. Patients with botulism, myasthenic syndrome, hypocalcemia, and hypomagnesemia have defects in transmitter release. The first response is often of very low amplitude, but successive stimuli evoke progressively larger responses. The response is not only facilitated by repetitive stimulation, but also by sustained exercise. The incremental response is somewhat greater with myasthenic syndrome than with botulism. Myasthenia gravis may produce an incremental response with repetitive stimulation at fast rates; however, the magnitude of the increment is usually limited.

Paired Stimulation

The response to paired stimuli can be abnormal in any disorder of neuromuscular transmission. However, the technique is predominantly used for diagnosis of presynaptic defects, such as botulism and myasthenic syndrome.

Physiology

A single stimulus gives a reproducible CMAP. If a second stimulus is given after the first, the CMAP is usually smaller if the interval between stimuli is short. This is because the second stimulus arrives within the refractory period of some of the muscle fibers (Figure 22.2). The second response usually disappears when the interval falls below 5 ms.

In presynaptic disorders, the second stimulus may produce a larger CMAP than the first for two reasons. First, release mechanisms are "primed," probably due to increased availability of calcium. Since more transmitter is released, the second stimulus may activate some muscle fibers that the first did not. Second, if a muscle fiber did not reach threshold, the end-plate potential likely has not completely decayed when the second arrives. Summation of the end-plate potentials can bring the muscle fiber membrane to threshold. The result is that the second CMAP is greater than the first.

Methods

Electrodes are placed as described for repetitive stimulation. Stimuli are given with variable interstimulus intervals. There is no uniformly agreed-upon protocol, but it is reasonable to start at an interstimulus interval of 15 ms and gradually reduce the interval. The most helpful data is obtained with interstimulus intervals of 5 to 10 ms.

The amplitude of the CMAP obtained in response to the first and second stimuli of each pair is measured. The ratio of the two responses is used for interpretation.

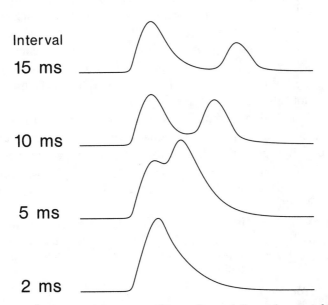

Figure 22.2 Paired stimulation. Paired stimuli are delivered at variable interstimulus intervals. The responses are recorded, and the amplitude to the first and second responses measured. No facilitation is normal. Facilitation of the second response is a positive result.

Interpretation

The normal response is for the second CMAP to be smaller than the first. With shorter interstimulus intervals, the second response becomes smaller and eventually disappears, usually at or below 5 ms. An abnormal response results in a larger second response at interstimulus intervals of 5 to 10 ms. Abnormal paired stimulation is consistent with a diagnosis of botulism or myasthenic syndrome; however, it is not diagnostic.

Single-Fiber Electromyography

Single-fiber EMG (SFEMG) is a time-consuming study used predominantly for the diagnosis of myasthenia gravis. False positives occur. Many clinicians feel that the cost-benefit ratio of the test is not satisfactory in a busy practice. The two main studies performed during SFEMG are jitter analysis and fiber density determination.

Jitter Analysis

Physiology

Single muscle fibers do not discharge exactly synchronously in creating a MUP. There may be several milliseconds difference in time of activation. This is termed the *interpotential interval* (IPI). The IPI for two muscle fibers, normally less than 4 ms, is very reproducible from discharge to discharge. The normal variation is less than 50 µs. Disorders of neuromuscular transmission may increase the variation because synaptic transmission is less secure, that is, the end-plate potential (EPP) is smaller, so that the muscle fiber action potential is higher on the hump of the EPP (see Figure 22.3). The time to threshold after the EPP is more variable.

The term *jitter* is derived from the appearance of the potentials on the oscilloscope display. The display is set so that the sweep is triggered by the first muscle fiber action potential. The second muscle fiber action potential appears a few milliseconds after the first. Since the first action potential is fixed in position on the display by the triggering apparatus, the second "jitters" back and forth as the IPI varies slightly.

Blocking is failure of discharge of either the first or second potential. This is due to the muscle fiber's EPP not reaching threshold. Disorders of neuromuscular transmission may not only result in increased jitter but also blocking.

Methods

The electrode is inserted into the muscle in the region of highest end-plate density. The extensor digitorum communis (EDC) is the most commonly studied muscle. After insertion of the electrode, the patient is asked to make a mild contraction, in the case of the EDC, extension of the

Normal Jitter

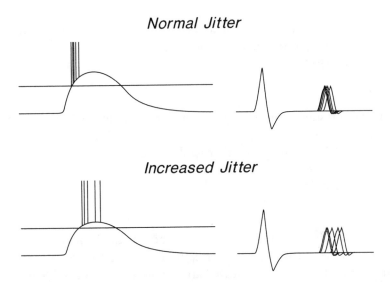

Increased Jitter

Figure 22.3   Physiological basis for jitter on single-fiber EMG. Left side is an intracellular recording after nerve stimulation.

middle finger (digit 3). The examiner wants to record potentials from two muscle fibers of one motor unit. The action potentials can be defined as being from one unit if there is an almost perfect time-lock between activation of the two fibers.

A pair is accepted if the following criteria are met:

- Muscle fibers are clearly of the same motor unit
- Rise time is less than 300 ms
- Amplitude is greater than 200 µV
- IPI is greater than 150 µs.

Measurements are made from the beginning of the upstroke of the potentials. This is best accomplished by using a computer to make direct measurement of the mean consecutive differences (MCD) of the IPIs. The IPIs of consecutive discharges are subtracted, and the absolute values stored. The sum of these absolute values is divided by the number of trials to give the MCD. The MCD is more accurate than the standard deviation of the IPI, since the MCD is a more direct index of discharge-to-discharge variation.

A second method of jitter determination is possible without a computer. Ten consecutive discharge pairs are superimposed on the oscilloscope screen or on photographic paper. Because of the triggering, the first potentials should be exactly superimposed, as above. The second potentials will occur within an expected range. The range of IPI variation is the time from takeoff of the earliest of the second potentials to the takeoff of the last of the second potentials. This is termed the R_{10} (for Range of 10 pairs). The R_{10} is determined for five electrode positions in the muscle and the mean R_{10} range calculated (MR_{10}). For that muscle, an estimated MCD is calculated from the following formula (Ekstedt et al. 1974):

$$MCD = MR_{10} * 0.37.$$

This formula results in an accurate estimation of the true MCD, which would have been calculated directly.

Jitter analysis involves not only calculation of variation of IPI but also the number of failures of conduction. This is termed *blocking*. Normal individuals have no blocking.

Interpretation

The mean consecutive difference should be less than 55 μs for EDC, the muscle usually studied. Normative data is available for other muscles. A normal muscle may have increased jitter in one of twenty muscle fiber pairs, but increased jitter or blocking in two or more of twenty pairs is abnormal. The findings are not subtle. Most patients with generalized myasthenia have greatly increased jitter in a large proportion of pairs. Patients with ocular myasthenia may have increased jitter only in facial muscles.

Jitter analysis is a more sensitive test than repetitive stimulation to detect disorders of neuromuscular transmission. For example, patients with myasthenia gravis often have increased jitter in clinically unaffected muscles. Normal jitter in a clinically weak muscle is strong evidence against the diagnosis of myasthenia.

Increased jitter can be seen in partially denervated muscles as well as in disorders of neuromuscular transmission. Chronic exercise may also increase jitter in otherwise normal individuals, probably due to mild denervation and reinnervation.

Blocking is a more specific sign of neuromuscular transmission disorders and is seldom seen in normal individuals. Some individuals 50 years or older may have blocking due to motor unit reorganization. Jitter is not significantly increased with age. In myasthenia gravis, blocking always occurs in the setting of increased jitter.

Fiber Density Determination

Fiber density is used to document chronic denervation. Increased fiber density is a sign of local reinnervation of denervated muscle fibers.

Physiology

Muscle fibers innervated by a single motor axon are scattered widely through a muscle; often only one muscle fiber is innervated by a single motor unit within a 300-micron radius. Fiber density is increased in patients with axonal neuropathies because denervated muscle fibers are reinnervated by sprouts from nearby surviving motor axons.

Methods

A SFEMG electrode is used, as described for jitter analysis. The needle is inserted into the muscle, the patient is asked to make a mild contraction, and a single muscle fiber action potential is recorded. A potential meets criteria for study if it has an amplitude of at least 200 μV and a rise time of less than 300 μs. When a potential is isolated, the clinical neurophysiologist looks for other muscle fiber action potentials that are part of the same motor unit. A muscle fiber action potential is classified as being part of the same motor unit if it occurs reproducibly in the same time relation to the first muscle fiber action potential. The secondary potential must also be at least 200 μV in amplitude with a rise time of less than 300 μs. This ensures that the potentials are within a 300-micron radius.

If the index potential is the only one identified in that motor unit, that electrode position has a fiber density of 1.0. If there are three muscle fiber potentials meeting criteria, the fiber density is 3.0. The fiber density is determined for at least twenty locations within the muscle and averaged across all examined locations. The muscle fiber density is expressed as a grand mean.

Interpretation

Normal values for fiber density are shown in Table 22.1. Increased fiber density indicates partial denervation and local reinnervation. Young children may have increased fiber density in the absence of neuromuscular disease.

Table 22.1 Normal Data for Fiber-Density Determination

	Age (years)			
Muscle	*10–25*	*26–50*	*50–75*	*>75*
Extensor digitorum communis	1.87	1.89	2.00	3.155
First dorsal interosseus	1.66	1.79	ID	ID
Tibialis anterior	2.12	2.11	2.07	ID

ID = Insufficient data.

Note: Upper limits of normal, calculated as mean ±2.5 standard deviations from the mean. All data are in milliseconds (ms).

23

□ □ □
□ □ □
□ □ □

Evaluation of Common Neuromuscular Problems

Electrophysiological testing is designed to answer specific clinical questions. The first task is to localize the site of the lesion. For this, Table 23.1 shows the expected nerve-conduction velocity (NCV) and electromyographic (EMG) findings with different lesions sites in the nerve-muscle axis. Table 23.2 presents a suggested evaluation of patients with specific complaints. Table 23.3 shows the NCV and EMG findings in common specific disorders. The following are recommendations on studies to choose for several common clinical questions.

General Questions

Peripheral Neuropathy

Peripheral neuropathies have a predominantly distal distribution and the longest nerves are the ones most likely affected. The following conduction studies are recommended as an initial screen:

- Tibial motor conduction
- Sural sensory conduction
- Tibial F wave.

If these studies are normal, the patient does not have a generalized demyelinating neuropathy.

Electromyography should be performed in distal muscles. Myopathies are occasionally mistaken for neuropathies, so proximal muscles should be studied as well, especially if nerve-conduction studies are normal. Ask the patient which movements are most impaired and study the muscles that perform those movements. If there are no localizing symptoms, and the request does not specify an area to study, then the tibialis anterior and rectus femoris

Table 23.1 Clinical Correlations of NCVs and EMG Findings

Axonal neuropathy
    NCV: Reduced CMAP amplitude, otherwise normal NCVs
    EMG: Acute and/or chronic denervation

Demyelinating neuropathy
    NCV: Slow motor and sensory NCVs
          Delayed F waves
    EMG: Usually normal EMG

Motor neuron degeneration
    NCV: Normal NCVs except possibly reduced CMAP amplitude
    EMG: Acute and chronic denervation

Sensory neuron degeneration
    NCV: Normal except possibly low SNAP amplitude
    EMG: Normal

Myopathy
    NCV: Normal. Occasionally low CMAP amplitude
    EMG: Myopathic findings

Neuromuscular transmission defect
    NCV: Normal or reduced CMAP amplitude
          Abnormal repetitive stimulation
          Abnormal response to paired stimulation
    EMG: Normal or mild denervation

NCV = Nerve-conduction velocities; EMG = Electromyography; CMAP = Compound motor action potential; SNAP = Sensory neural action potential.

should be examined. Some clinical neurophysiologists prefer to study the extensor digitorum brevis because of its very distal location. I disagree. The muscle belly is small and it is easy to insert the needle into a tendon or through the muscle into connective tissue.

Myopathy

Some clinical neurophysiologists perform EMG without NCVs when evaluating patients for myopathy. However, the observation of typical myopathic features on EMG does not exclude the existence of a concurrent neuropathy. At least one motor and sensory nerve conduction should be performed. For motor-conduction studies, I prefer to study the tibial nerve because the peroneal nerve is more susceptible to pressure palsies, especially when mobility is impaired by weakness. The sural nerve is preferred for sensory conduction studies because it is technically easier to study than the superficial peroneal.

Table 23.2 Recommended Evaluation of Common Neuromuscular Problems

Problem	NCV	EMG
Brachial plexopathy	Median motor NCV Median sensory NCV Median F wave	First dorsal interosseus Pronator teres Biceps Triceps
Carpal tunnel syndrome	Median motor NCV Median sensory NCV	Abductor pollicis brevis
Cervical radiculopathy	Median motor NCV Median sensory NCV Median F wave	Abductor pollicis brevis First dorsal interosseus Extensor digitorum communis Biceps Triceps Deltoid Cervical paraspinal muscles
Foot drop	Peroneal motor NCV Peroneal F wave	Tibialis anterior Peroneus longus Short head of biceps femoris
Lumbar plexopathy	Tibial motor NCV Peroneal motor NCV Sural sensory NCV Tibial F wave Peroneal F wave	Tibialis anterior Medial gastrocnemius Vastus medialis
Lumbar radiculopathy	Tibial motor NCV Sural sensory NCV Tibial F wave H reflex	Tibialis anterior Medial gastrocnemius Vastus medialis Lumbar paraspinal muscles
Meralgia paresthetica	Tibial motor NCV Sural sensory NCV Femoral distal latency	Rectus femoris Vastus medialis Tibialis anterior Medial gastrocnemius
Motoneuron disease	Tibial motor NCV Sural sensory NCV	Muscles in 3 nerve distributions in 3 extremities
Peripheral neuropathy	Tibial motor NCV Sural sensory NCV Tibial F wave	Tibialis anterior Medial gastrocnemius
Peroneal palsy	Peroneal motor NCV Sup. peroneal sensory NCV Peroneal F wave	Tibialis anterior Peroneus longus Short head of biceps femoris
Radial neuropathy	Radial motor NCV Radial sensory NCV	Extensor digitorum communis

Table 23.2 (continued)   Recommended Evaluation of Common Neuromuscular Problems

Problem	NCV	EMG
Sciatic neuropathy	Tibial motor NCV Peroneal motor NCV Sural sensory NCV Tibial F wave Peroneal F wave	Tibialis anterior Medial gastrocnemius Vastus medialis Gluteus medius
Spinal stenosis	*See* Lumbar radiculopathy	
Ulnar neuropathy	Ulnar motor NCV below elbow Ulnar motor NCV across elbow Ulnar sensory NCV	First dorsal interosseus
Tarsal tunnel syndrome	Medial plantar motor NCV Lateral plantar motor NCV	Abductor hallucis
Thoracic outlet syndrome	Median motor NCV Median sensory NCV Ulnar motor NCV Ulnar F wave	Abductor pollicis brevis First dorsal interosseus Extensor digitorum communis

NCV = Nerve-conduction velocity.

Note: These studies are recommended as minimum evaluation to look for the indicated disorder. In many cases, additional studies have to be done to localize the lesion. For example, if the recommended studies for carpal tunnel syndrome are abnormal, the ulnar and radial nerves should also be examined to differentiate between an isolated mononeuropathy versus a polyneuropathy or plexopathy. Also, the study should not be guided only by the requisition.

The EMG should be directed at weak muscles. If these show no abnormalities, additional muscles need not be examined. If they show myopathic changes, then clinically unaffected muscles should be studied to determine the extent of disease. Alternatively, if the muscles show neuropathic changes, the EMG study must be expanded to determine whether the denervation is from mononeuropathy, polyneuropathy, or motor-neuron disease. Additional nerve-conduction studies may be needed.

Vague Questions

Neurophysiologic studies should not be a substitute for neurologic consultation, but this is sometimes the case. Such patients usually have poorly defined reasons for the requested study, often due to poorly defined

Table 23.3 NCV and EMG Findings in Common Neuromuscular Disorders

Disorder	NCV	EMG
Amyotrophic lateral sclerosis	Decreased CMAP amplitude. Otherwise Nl NCVs.	Widespread denervation
Carpal tunnel syndrome	Increased median motor DL Decreased median sensory NCV	Denervation APB
Guillain-Barré syndrome	Increased F-wave latency Decreased motor and sensory NCV	Usually Nl. Occasional mild denervation.
Muscular dystrophy	± decreased CMAP amplitude. Otherwise Nl NCV.	Myo mainly in proximal muscles
Myasthenia gravis	Ab repetitive stimulation	± Fibs
Peroneal palsy	Decreased peroneal motor NCV Decreased peroneal CMAP amplitude	Denervation TA Nl Short head of biceps femoris
Polymyositis	± decreased CMAP amplitude. Otherwise Nl NCV.	Myo mainly in proximal muscles
Pronator teres syndrome	Decreased median motor NCV	Denervation APB Denervation FDS Nl Pronator teres
Radiculopathy	Usually Nl NCVs. Nl F waves.	Denervation in dermatomal distribution
Thoracic outlet syndrome	Decreased ulnar SNAP amplitude Increased ulnar F-wave latency	Denervation hand intrinsics including APB
Tarsal tunnel syndrome	Increased tibial motor DL Decreased NCV of medial or lateral planter n.	Denervation AHB
Ulnar neuropathy: Guyon's canal	Increased ulnar motor DL Decreased ulnar sensory NCV	Denervation FDI
Ulnar neuropathy: Cubital tunnel	Slow conduction across elbow	Denervation FDI, ADM, FDP

CMAP = Compound motor action potential; DL = Distal latency; EMG = Electromyography; Fibs = Fibrillation potentials and positive sharp waves; Myo = Myopathic features; NCV = Nerve-conduction velocity; Nl = Normal; SNAP = Sensory nerve action potential; ± = Plus or minus: may or may not be present but not a prominent feature.

Muscles: ADM = Abductor digiti minimi (quinti); AHB = Abductor hallucis brevis; APB = Abductor pollicis brevis; EDC = Extensor digitorum communis; FDI = First dorsal interosseus.

Note: Not all findings are diagnostic in all individuals with a particular disorder. Also, findings may not be specific, so alternative diagnoses need to be considered.

clinical data. If the clinical neurophysiologist cannot develop a sense of the problem by a brief history and physical examination, the following screening tests should be performed:

1. NCV:
   a. Tibial motor NCV
   b. Tibial F wave
   c. Sural sensory NCV
2. EMG:
   a. Tibialis anterior
   b. Rectus femoris

If all are normal, it is unlikely that the patient has a neuromuscular disease. The only generalized neuromuscular disorders that these studies might miss are neuromuscular transmission defects and rare motor neuronopathies. The impression may read: "Normal study. No evidence of generalized myopathy or neuropathy. If a specific disorder is suspected, additional studies may be helpful, and will be performed upon request."

Specific Questions

Recommended minimum NCS and EMG studies for specific clinical questions are presented in Table 23.2. If all of the recommended studies are normal, further examination is not indicated. If abnormalities support the diagnosis, other investigations may be needed. Refer to the chapters on specific disease processes for guidelines on additional studies to diagnose the disorders.

24 □ □ □
□ □ □
□ □ □

Disorders of Peripheral Nerve

The essentials of differential diagnosis of neuromuscular disorders was described in detail in chapter 19, "Basic Principles of Nerve-Conduction Studies and Electromyography." The most important information obtained from nerve-conduction studies (NCS) and electromyography (EMG) is location of the lesion and classification of lesion type. This section discusses electrophysiological features of some of the more important neuropathies. Clinical characteristics are not presented. Refer to standard neurology texts or especially the book by Dyck et al. (1984) for an excellent discussion of peripheral neuropathies.

Mononeuropathies

The hallmark of mononeuropathies is slowed conduction in an isolated nerve, reduced compound motor action potential (CMAP) and/or sensory neural action potential (SNAP) amplitude, and EMG signs of denervation in innervated muscles. Signs of denervation may not be seen if the lesion is minor or due to neurapraxia. Signs of acute denervation may not be present for three to four weeks. Therefore, a repeat study is indicated if the initial study was within four weeks from the onset of a mononeuropathy. Some studies must be done immediately, especially after trauma, to determine if the nerve is in continuity. The presence of only a few motor unit potentials is often reassuring to the clinician.

Median Nerve

Carpal Tunnel Syndrome
Carpal tunnel syndrome is the most common entrapment neuropathy. Motor and sensory conduction of the median nerve through the wrist is slowed, that is, motor distal latency is prolonged and sensory nerve-

conduction velocity (NCV) is slow. At least one of these measures is abnormal in more than 90% of patients with clinically diagnosed carpal tunnel syndrome. Median motor NCV between the arm and wrist is normal. F waves are normal.

The EMG of median-innervated muscles is usually normal; however, there may be signs of acute denervation when injury is severe. If acute denervation is present in the abductor pollicis brevis, at least one ulnar-innervated muscle should be examined (for example, first dorsal interosseus) to ensure that the lesion is not in the lower plexus (roots C8-T1). Also, more proximal median-innervated muscles should be examined to localize the lesion at the carpal tunnel rather than pronator teres or elsewhere. The most convenient muscles to examine are the flexor digitorum superficialis and the radial half of the flexor digitorum profundus. These should be normal.

Pronator Teres Syndrome

The median nerve is compressed as it passes through the pronator teres in the proximal forearm. Median motor NCV through the forearm is slow but the distal latency is normal. Sensory NCV is normal because the segment tested is distal to the pronator teres.

The EMG usually shows acute and chronic denervation of the abductor pollicis brevis, flexor digitorum superficialis, and median-innervated portion of the flexor digitorum profundus. The pronator teres is not denervated, because it is innervated proximal to the site of compression. This is an important feature that distinguishes the pronator teres syndrome from compression of the median nerve by the ligament of Struthers.

Compression by the Ligament of Struthers

The ligament of Struthers is a fibrous band above the medial epicondyle. The clinical syndrome of median nerve compression by the ligament of Struthers resembles the pronator teres syndrome. Most median-innervated muscles of the forearm are weak. The differentiating feature is involvement of the pronator teres. In pronator teres syndrome, the pronator teres is tender but its strength is normal and there is no denervation on EMG. When median nerve compression occurs at the ligament of Struthers, the pronator teres is weak and shows acute and chronic denervation on EMG. Other neurophysiologic findings are as described for the pronator teres syndrome.

Anterior Interosseus Syndrome

The anterior interosseus nerve is a branch of the median nerve that innervates several muscles in the forearm, including the flexor digitorum profundus of the first two digits, flexor pollicis longus, and pronator quadratus. This syndrome is caused by injury of the nerve after it leaves the main trunk of the median nerve. Nerve-conduction velocities are usually normal. Stimulation of the anterior interosseus nerve at the elbow may reveal increased distal latency of the CMAP recorded from the pronator quadratus. The EMG shows denervation in the flexor pollicis longus, median-innervated portion of the flexor digitorum profundus, and pronator quadratus.

Ulnar Nerve

The most common locations for lesion of the ulnar nerve are at Guyon's canal and near the elbow. Many diabetics show wasting and denervation in the ulnar-innervated intrinsic muscles of the hands. These patients have a prominent ulnar neuropathy, superimposed on a more generalized polyneuropathy.

Entrapment at Guyon's Canal
The ulnar nerve passes from the forearm into the hand through Guyon's canal. Ulnar compression at the wrist is analogous to the carpal tunnel syndrome. Unlike compression of the ulnar nerve at the elbow, the ulnar-innervated flexors in the forearm are unaffected and the sensory loss is confined to the ulnar side of the hand, sparing the forearm.

Ulnar NCVs are slowed across the wrist, and the distal latency is increased when recording from the abductor digiti minimi. The EMG shows denervation of the abductor digiti minimi and first dorsal interosseus but a normal pattern in the flexor digitorum profundus and flexor carpi ulnaris.

Entrapment Near the Elbow
The ulnar nerve is especially susceptible to injury as it crosses under the medial epicondyle of the humerus. Ulnar motor NCV is slow across the elbow but usually normal in the forearm. The difference in NCV should exceed 10 meters per second (10 m/s) to be significant. The CMAP is reduced in amplitude if the nerve damage is severe; SNAPs are often absent or very small in amplitude. Stimulation can be performed at measured intervals across the cubital tunnel for precise localization.

The EMG shows acute and chronic denervation of the ulnar-innervated intrinsic muscles of the hand and the ulnar-innervated portion of the flexor digitorum profundus. The flexor carpi ulnaris is not denervated, because its innervation leaves the main ulnar nerve proximal to the elbow.

Lesion of the Palmar Branch of the Ulnar Nerve
Pressure on the palmar branch of the ulnar nerve can produce damage after the innervation to the abductor digiti minimi and digit 5 has already taken off. Therefore, routine motor and sensory NCVs are normal, including motor distal latency. Distal latency to the first dorsal interosseus is

prolonged, and denervation is seen in this muscle. The superficial sensory branch of the ulnar nerve may be damaged, especially in bicycle riders.

Radial Nerve

The most common sites of injury to the radial nerve are at the spiral groove and in the forearm, as the nerve penetrates the supinator muscle. Less common sites are the elbow with radius dislocation, the wrist from handcuffs, and damage to the recurrent epicondylar branch (one form of "tennis elbow").

Compression at the Spiral Groove

Nerve conduction across the spiral groove is slow. The CMAPs and SNAPs are absent if the lesion is complete. With severe but incomplete lesions, the distal latency of the CMAP may be prolonged and distal conduction studies slowed.

The EMG shows acute and chronic denervation of all radial-innervated finger and wrist extensors. Proximal lesions cause denervation of the triceps as well. It is important to determine if any motor units can be activated by attempted voluntary contraction. The presence of motor units indicates that the nerve is in continuity and there is a better prognosis for recovery.

Posterior Interosseus Syndrome

As the radial nerve enters the forearm, it divides into the posterior interosseus nerve and a superficial sensory branch. The posterior interosseus nerve supplies the finger and wrist extensors. Injuries to the nerve cause weakness without sensory loss.

Nerve conduction is slowed through the involved segment. The EMG shows denervation in the wrist and finger extensors, with sparing of the extensor carpi radialis longus and the supinator. Both muscles are innervated by branches that arise proximal to the lesion.

Brachial Plexus Lesions

Upper Plexus Lesion (Erb's Palsy)

Proximal muscles are more affected than distal muscles and intrinsic muscles of the hand are spared. The most prominent denervation is in the deltoid, biceps, supraspinatus, and infraspinatus. The serratus anterior and rhomboids are spared, because their innervation is proximal to the lesion.

Lower Plexus Lesion

The lower brachial plexus is susceptible to trauma, but is especially sensitive to neoplastic infiltration. Tumors arising from the apex of the lung will produce infiltration and/or compression of the lower plexus. Denervation is most prominent in muscles innervated by the median and ulnar nerves (roots C8-T1).

Neoplastic infiltration is differentiated from radiation plexopathy mainly on clinical grounds; however, NCS and EMG can be helpful. Tumor infiltration usually slows conduction through the plexus, while conduction is usually normal in radiation plexopathy. The EMG shows myokymia in many patients with radiation plexopathy, but not in patients with neoplastic infiltration.

Idiopathic Brachial Plexitis

Nerve-conduction velocities may be normal or show slowing through the plexus. Severe lesions may cause slowing of distal median and ulnar conduction. The EMG may show denervation not only in weak muscles but also in muscles that seem clinically unaffected. However, sufficient time must elapse before the EMG is abnormal. In practice, EMG shows denervation at about the time that the patient has developed significant weakness. Therefore, if there is pain but no weakness, the initial EMG may be normal and a later study may be more revealing.

Peroneal Neuropathy

Peroneal pressure palsy occurs most commonly at the fibular neck. Peroneal palsy is diagnosed by slowed NCV of the peroneal nerve across the fibular neck or reduced amplitude of the CMAP when stimulating above the lesion site. Denervation is seen in the tibialis anterior and peroneii; however, there is no denervation in the short head of the biceps femoris. This latter muscle is innervated by a branch of the peroneal division which takes off proximal to the fibular neck.

Slowing across the fibular neck is significant if it is at least 10 m/sec slower than distal conduction velocity. Amplitude difference is significant if the response to proximal stimulation is at least 25% less than the response to distal stimulation.

Occasionally, sciatic nerve lesions may be misdiagnosed as peroneal palsy. The peroneal division of the sciatic nerve is more susceptible to damage than the tibial division. Abnormalities in the tibial distribution may be subtle. Therefore, it is important to study some tibial-innervated muscles, even in cases of relatively "pure" peroneal palsy.

Tibial Neuropathy

Tibial nerve entrapment behind the medial malleolus is called *tarsal tunnel syndrome*. It is relatively uncommon. The motor distal latency of the medial or lateral plantar nerve is increased. In order to test the medial plantar nerve, recording is made from the abductor hallucis; for the lateral plantar nerve, recording is made from the abductor digiti quinti.

Some neurophysiologists use incremental stimulation through the tarsal tunnel, similar to that performed for carpal tunnel syndrome. However, this probably does not add anything to careful measurement of medial and lateral plantar nerve distal latency.

Sciatic Nerve Lesions

Piriformis Syndrome

Piriformis syndrome is compression of the sciatic nerve by the piriformis muscle. It is a clinical diagnosis with no unique electrophysiological findings. Denervation in the distribution of the peroneal division of the sciatic nerve, with lesser or no involvement of muscles innervated by the tibial division is the only EMG finding. Denervation of distal muscles with sparing of the gluteus medius is supportive of piriformis syndrome, since this muscle receives innervation from a branch of the sciatic which arises proximal to the lesion. Piriformis syndrome is differentiated from peroneal neuropathy at the fibula by involvement of the short head of the biceps femoris in the former, but not the latter. The innervation of this muscle is proximal to the popliteal fossa.

Sciatic Stretch

The lithotomy position (extension, abduction, and slight flexion of the legs) is used in many surgical procedures. This position stretches the sciatic nerve as it passes through the sciatic notch into the leg. The patient awakens from anesthesia with weakness of sciatic-innervated muscles. We have also seen this syndrome in patients who sustained sudden forward flexion at the waist.

Tibial motor and sural sensory NCVs are typically normal; however, there may be increased tibial F-wave latency. The EMG is normal or shows only a decreased number of motor units immediately after injury.

Mononeuropathy Multiplex

Diabetes mellitus and polyarteritis nodosa are the most common disorders that cause mononeuritis multiplex in the United States. Leprosy is the most common cause worldwide.

Polyarteritis Nodosa

Polyarteritis nodosa is an idiopathic connective tissue disorder characterized by multifocal vasculitis. This is a clinical diagnosis and can be supported but not confirmed by electrophysiological studies.

Affected nerves show slowed or blocked conduction at the site of arteritis, and EMG shows acute and chronic denervation in affected areas. Complete denervation causes fibrillation potentials and positive sharp waves, and absence of motor unit activation with attempted voluntary effort.

Leprosy

Leprosy is probably one of the most common causes of neuropathy worldwide. The neuropathy is caused by either primary nerve infiltration or by infarction of the vaso nervorum.

Nerve conduction in the involved regions of the nerves are blocked or slowed. The EMG shows acute and chronic denervation in muscles innervated by involved nerves. If the neuropathy is predominantly due to cutaneous vasculitis, only the distal sensory branches may be involved.

Polyneuropathies

Demyelinating Neuropathies

Guillain-Barré Syndrome

Motor and sensory NCV studies of the upper and lower limbs may be normal early in the course but later are slowed. The earliest changes are prolongation or absence of the F wave and dispersion of the CMAP. Electromyographic evidence of denervation is unusual but may develop in severe cases. Polyphasic potentials and reduced recruitment are seen later in the course.

When demyelination is severe, permanent axonal loss may occur in distal muscles. The EMG and NCV usually return to normal, but conduction slowing may persist in severe cases.

Chronic Inflammatory Demyelinating Polyneuropathy

With chronic inflammatory demyelinating polyneuropathy (CIDP), the first electrophysiological abnormality is slowing of the F wave. Motor and sensory NCVs of the upper and lower extremities slow subsequently. EMG is normal in the first weeks of disease but later shows widespread denervation. The denervation is typically a mixture of acute and chronic findings: fibrillation potentials, positive sharp waves, and high-amplitude long-duration polyphasic motor unit potentials.

Although patients often clinically improve, NCVs usually remain slow. I have not found serial NCVs to be helpful for following patients with CIDP.

Axonal Neuropathies

Toxic Neuropathies

Most toxic neuropathies cause axonal degenerations, but demyelination is occasionally seen. The compounds that most often cause neuropathy are vincristine, cisplatin, lead, and ethanol. There are no specific findings on NCV and EMG to differentiate between toxic axonal neuropathies and other causes of axonal neuropathy.

Neuronal Degenerations

Amyotrophic Lateral Sclerosis

Amyotrophic Lateral Sclerosis (ALS) is the most common neuronal degeneration. Both upper and lower motoneurons degenerate. Motor and sensory NCVs are normal, although CMAP may be of reduced amplitude. The EMG shows widespread denervation. A screening examination for motoneuron disease should include examination of at least three muscles in different nerve distributions in each of three limbs. The head may be substituted for one limb. Features of both acute and chronic denervation are typical, but acute changes may be mild as the disease progresses. Fasciculations are common in ALS, but fasciculations in the absence of other clinical or electrophysiological abnormalities do not make the diagnosis. Fasciculations occur in other, less serious disorders and in some normal individuals.

Spinal Muscular Atrophy

Motor NCVs in spinal muscular atrophies are normal or only mildly slowed. Sensory NCVs are normal. The EMG shows prominent denervation, with fibrillation potentials and positive sharp waves. Recruitment may be incomplete, with rapid firing of single units. Long-duration polyphasic motor unit potentials (neuropathic motor units) are rare early in the disease but then become very prominent with ongoing motor unit reorganization.

Poliomyelitis

Poliomyelitis is caused by a neurotropic enterovirus that destroys anterior horn cells. Motor NCVs are normal or near normal. EMG shows chronic denervation. Since poliomyelitis is focal or multifocal, the EMG findings are most prominent in muscles that are clinically involved.

Selected Neuropathies

Several major classes of neuropathy do not fall clearly within the above categories. We will now review the most important classes.

Diabetic Neuropathy

Diabetes mellitus is the cause of four different neuropathies:

- Small-fiber polyneuropathy
- Large-fiber polyneuropathy

- Autonomic neuropathy
- Mononeuropathy and mononeuropathy multiplex.

The small-fiber neuropathy is a distal predominantly sensory neuropathy. C-fiber dysfunction predominates, although axonal degeneration also involves motor fibers. Nerve-conduction velocity studies may be normal, because compound action potentials are mediated by large myelinated fibers; EMG is usually normal as well. The most sensitive test of small fiber dysfunction is the sympathetic skin response.

The large-fiber neuropathy involves both motor and sensory axons, with particular loss of fibers subserving motor function, vibration, joint perception, and two-point discrimination. Autonomic neuropathy is also a predominantly small fiber disorder and is a common feature of all diabetic neuropathies. Mononeuropathy can affect one or several nerves (mononeuropathy multiplex). Mononeuropathy multiplex is diagnosed by finding multifocal NCV and/or EMG changes. The most commonly affected nerves are femoral, lumbosacral plexus, oculomotor, abducens, ulnar, and median, but any cranial nerves may be affected. Mononeuropathy of the femoral nerve or proximal lumbar plexus is often termed *diabetic amyotrophy*. Mononeuropathy affecting individual spinal roots is termed *diabetic radiculopathy*.

Nerve conduction is slowed in most patients with diabetic neuropathy, even though the demyelination is often secondary to axonal degeneration. The EMG usually shows denervation in clinically affected muscles.

Hereditary Neuropathies

Hereditary Motor-Sensory Neuropathy Type I

Hereditary motor-sensory neuropathy type I (HMSN-I) is the demyelinating or hypertrophic form of Charcot-Marie-Tooth disease. Motor and sensory NCVs are slow, often to 20 to 30 m/sec, and distal motor latencies are prolonged. F waves are absent or delayed. The EMG may suggest mild denervation, but the features of axonal degeneration are much less prominent than the features of demyelination. Slowing of nerve conduction may involve the facial nerve causing an abnormal blink reflex.

Hereditary Motor-Sensory Neuropathy Type II

Hereditary motor-sensory neuropathy type II (HMSN-II) is the neuronal form of Charcot-Marie-Tooth disease. It is clinically similar to HMSN-I; however, the NCV and EMG findings are very different. Motor and sensory NCVs are either normal or mildly slow, indicating relative preservation of myelin. Motor distal latency may be increased, and CMAP and SNAP amplitudes reduced. The EMG shows signs of acute and chronic denervation, including prominent fibrillation potentials, fasciculations, and high-amplitude long-duration polyphasic motor unit potentials.

Hereditary Motor-Sensory Neuropathy Type III

Hereditary motor-sensory neuropathy type III (HMSN-III) is Déjérine-Sottas disease. It is a demyelinating condition clinically similar to HMSN-I but distinguished by inheritance and severity of disease. Motor and sensory conduction velocities are slow, and motor distal latencies are increased because of demyelination of distal nerve segments. Denervation changes on EMG are not as prominent as are the slowed nerve-conduction velocities.

A focal form of HMSN-III has been described. Only one nerve is affected. Nerve-conduction velocities in other nerves are normal. The EMG is normal except for in the distribution of the affected nerve, where there is prominent acute and chronic denervation.

Hereditary Motor-Sensory Neuropathy Type IV

Hereditary motor-sensory neuropathy type IV (HMSN-IV) is Refsum's disease, with both central and peripheral nervous system involvement. In the peripheral nervous system, demyelination causes slowed conduction velocities. Degeneration of anterior horn cells causes EMG features of acute and chronic denervation.

Hereditary Motor-Sensory Neuropathy Type V

Hereditary motor-sensory neuropathy type V (HMSN-V) is the combination of peripheral neuropathy plus upper motor neuron degeneration. The electrophysiological changes are similar to HMSN-IV, and the two are distinguished by clinical features.

Friedreich's Ataxia

This is a hereditary ataxia transmitted by autosomal recessive inheritance. There are clinical and electrophysiological features of peripheral neuropathy. Motor NCVs are usually normal but SNAPs are absent or of low amplitude. If a SNAP is obtainable, NCV is normal or only mildly slowed, because the sensory defect is due to sensory neuron degeneration.

25 □ □ □
□ □ □
□ □ □

Disorders of Muscle

The major categories of muscle disease are dystrophies, inflammatory myopathies, and metabolic myopathies (endocrine, genetic, and toxic).

Motor and sensory conduction velocities are normal. Compound motor action potential (CMAP) amplitude may be reduced because muscle fibers fail to be activated. Electromyography (EMG) is informative. Insertion may elicit complex repetitive discharges. At rest, there are fibrillation potentials and positive sharp waves. Motor unit potentials (MUPs) are reduced in amplitude and brief in duration. With increasing effort, units are recruited earlier than normal because of reduced tension output of the muscle fibers ("early recruitment").

Muscular Dystrophies

Limb-girdle dystrophy is the common phenotypic expression of several disorders. Many of the male patients diagnosed as limb-girdle dystrophy have Becker's dystrophy, some may have a neuropathic disorder, and others have a metabolic myopathy. The EMG shows myopathic features in the majority of patients. Those with neuropathic features probably have a spinal muscular atrophy.

Duchenne and Becker's muscular dystrophy are characterized by normal NCVs. The EMG shows fibrillation potentials, complex repetitive discharges, and early recruitment. Fibrillation potentials are not as common as in inflammatory myopathies and denervation. Toward the end of the disease, muscle is replaced by fat and connective tissue and insertional activity is reduced or absent.

Myotonic dystrophy is characterized by myotonia on EMG. Myotonia is the repetitive discharge of muscle fibers with an initially high frequency that gradually declines. This gives a "dive-bomber" sound in the audio monitor. Myopathic MUPs may also be seen. Occasional neuropathic features include slow motor conduction and a reduced number of functioning motor units.

Fascio-scapulo-humeral (FSH) dystrophy or "syndrome" is an autosomal dominant disorder characterized by progressive weakness of the face and shoulder girdle. Scapulo-peroneal dystrophy or "syndrome" is probably a variant phenotype of the same genetic disorder. The EMG may be normal in mild or early cases. Typical findings are myopathic MUPs and early recruitment. Fibrillation potentials are occasionally seen but are not prominent. Neuropathic changes are seen both by electrophysiological and histologic studies in some patients, suggesting that this is a neuropathic disorder rather than a dystrophy.

Inflammatory Myopathies

The electrophysiological changes in all inflammatory myopathies are essentially the same. Nerve-conduction velocities are normal, although the CMAP amplitude may be reduced. The typical EMG findings are fibrillation potentials and positive sharp waves, myopathic MUPs, and complex repetitive discharges. Fibrillation potentials are more common in inflammatory myopathies than in muscular dystrophies. Abnormalities are more prominent in clinically weak muscles. The EMG is normal in approximately 10% of patients with typical polymyositis. This may be due to sampling error or to periods of relative inactivity during the course of the disease.

Metabolic Myopathies

Mitochondrial disorders may present as neuropathy or myopathy. Therefore, NCV and EMG should both be done when a mitochondrial myopathy is suspected. Tibial motor conduction and sural sensory NCV are a sufficient screen. If the sural sensory neural action potential (SNAP) is absent with a normal tibial motor NCV, a sensory NCV in the arm or superficial peroneal sensory NCV should be performed.

Endocrine myopathies may be associated with the following disorders:

- Cushing's syndrome
- Addison's disease
- Thyrotoxicosis
- Hypothyroidism (rarely)
- Hyperparathyroidism (rarely).

NCVs are normal except in hypothyroidism, in which case they may be slowed. EMG may show minor myopathic features in all of these disorders.

Steroid myopathy (Cushing's syndrome) is a clinical diagnosis. The EMG usually does not show myopathic features. The NCVs are also normal, although CMAP amplitude may be reduced.

Carnitine palmityl transferase deficiency usually has normal NCV and EMG findings. Patients with Carnitine deficiency have myopathic findings with small-amplitude polyphasic MUPs. Fibrillation potentials are seen but are rare.

Syndromes of Continuous Muscle Fiber Activity

Disorders of increased muscle fiber activity are classified into the following categories depending on the site of defect:

- Tetanus
- Stiff-man syndrome
- Schwartz-Jampel syndrome
- Neuromyotonia (Isaac's syndrome).

Tetanus is characterized by involuntary discharge of motor units. The toxin works at the spinal level, blocking postsynaptic inhibition, thereby increasing the excitability of motoneurons. The EMG shows repetitive MUPs that are abolished by peripheral nerve or neuromuscular block. The discharges are attenuated during sleep and with general or spinal anesthesia.

Stiff-man syndrome is not really a disorder of muscle; it is due to excessive motoneuron activation. The reason for the enhanced discharge is unknown. Excessive motor unit activity results in involuntary muscle contraction involving predominantly proximal muscles. Affected muscles show normal MUPs with coactivation of agonists and antagonists. Discharges are attenuated by sleep, general anesthesia, benzodiazepines, peripheral nerve block, or neuromuscular block.

Schwartz-Jampel syndrome is characterized by multiple congenital anomalies in association with increased muscle fiber activity. The defect is probably at the nerve terminal. Clinically, the muscle activity looks like myotonia, but on EMG the discharges have the appearance of complex repetitive discharges, lacking the frequency modulation of true myotonia. The discharges are abolished by neuromuscular block, but not by nerve block.

The term *neuromyotonia* is designed to differentiate these discharges from myotonia of primary muscle origin, as in myotonic dystrophy. Neuromyotonia differs from Stiff-man syndrome in that the EMG shows continuous activity of single muscle fibers rather than complete motor units. The muscle fibers discharge repetitively at frequencies that are initially high and gradually decline. This is similar to true myotonia, but the discharges have an invariant decline in frequency rather than a waxing and waning frequency. Also, these discharges are apparent at rest while myotonia is evoked prominently by insertion. The amplitude of MUPs may be reduced because of loss of functioning muscle fibers due to continuous activity. The defect is probably in the terminal motor axon. Therefore, the discharges are abolished by neuromuscular block, but not by peripheral nerve block, spinal block, or general anesthesia.

Miscellaneous Disorders of Muscle

Myotonia congenita is usually characterized by normal NCVs, but myotonia on the EMG. Repetitive stimulation produces a decremental response. The decrement is greater with high frequencies of stimulation.

Paramyotonia congenita is characterized by myotonia that worsens with exercise or exposure to cold. The NCVs are normal. Repetitive stimulation often results in a decremental response.

The periodic paralyses are a family of disorders all characterized by abnormal loss of excitability of the muscle fiber membrane. Between attacks NCVs are normal. The EMG is often normal but may show some myopathic features, indicating a myopathy. During an attack, motor nerve stimulation activates fewer muscle fibers. Therefore the CMAP is smaller. Myotonia may be seen in hyperkalemic periodic paralysis, blurring the distinction between this entity and paramyotonia congenita.

26 ▢▢▢ ▢▢▢ ▢▢▢

Disorders of Neuromuscular Transmission

Disorders of neuromuscular transmission typically produce abnormalities on repetitive stimulation, paired stimuli, and single-fiber electromyography (EMG) testing. However, similar abnormalities are occasionally seen in peripheral neuropathies and motor neuronopathies.

Repetitive stimulation and single-fiber EMG are performed on patients who are being evaluated for the possibility of myasthenia gravis. Paired stimuli are performed mainly for botulism. Myasthenic syndrome is associated with abnormalities on both repetitive stimulation and single-fiber testing.

Myasthenia Gravis

Myasthenia gravis is due to failure of neuromuscular transmission. Antibodies bind to the acetylcholine receptor on the postsynaptic membrane. This binding stimulates internalization and degradation of the receptor. Therefore, there are fewer receptors available for binding with acetylcholine. When an action potential depolarizes the presynaptic membrane, the transmitter cannot activate enough receptors to evoke an action potential in the muscle fiber. The sarcolemmal depolarization is insufficient.

Sensory conduction studies are normal, as are motor NCVs, but the amplitude of the CMAP may be reduced. Repetitive stimulation results in a decremental response.

The EMG is usually normal. The amplitudes of the motor unit potentials (MUPs) may fluctuate. Occasional myopathic MUPs may be seen but not fibrillation potentials and long-duration polyphasics. Single-fiber electromyography shows increased jitter.

The constellation of neurodiagnostic findings must be considered together. Increased jitter and variable MUP amplitude can be observed with denervating diseases. Signs of active and chronic denervation should be notably absent for a diagnosis of myasthenia gravis.

Neonatal Myasthenic Syndromes

A new classification of neonatal myasthenic syndromes was recently presented by Misulis and Fenichel (1989). The classification is based on pathophysiology (see Table 26.1). Diagnosis of these syndromes depends on techniques not readily available in most laboratories, for example, muscle acetylcholinesterase assay, in vitro intracellular electrophysiology, receptor binding studies. Most laboratories can narrow the differential diagnosis by clinical examination. Repetitive stimulation is usually not helpful, because it is abnormal in virtually all patients with genetic myasthenia. Normal repetitive stimulation responses at 3 Hz have been reported in some patients with impaired acetylcholine receptor function.

Acetylcholinesterase deficiency and slow-channel syndrome are characterized by repetitive discharge of muscle fibers by a single neural stimulus. A motor nerve is stimulated in the usual manner. A needle electrode is placed

Table 26.1   Neonatal Myasthenia

Genetic
1. Presynaptic
   a. Abnormal ACh resynthesis or mobilization
   b. Abnormal ACh release
2. Postsynaptic
   a. End-plate AChE deficiency
   b. Reduced number of AChRs
   c. Impaired function of AChRs
   d. Slow-channel syndrome
Acquired
1. AChR antibody positive
   a. Transitory neonatal
   b. Juvenile myasthenia
     i. Generalized
     ii. Mainly ocular
2. AChR antibody negative
   a. Juvenile myasthenia
     i. Mainly ocular
     ii. Relapsing ocular

ACh = Acetylcholine; AChE = Acetylcholinesterase; AChR = Acetylcholine receptor.

Note: Antibody-negative juvenile myasthenia may occur in individuals who are genetically predisposed.

Source: Adapted with permission from Misulis and Fenichel. Genetic forms of myasthenia gravis, K. Swaman, ed. *Pediatric Neurology* 5 (1989):205–10.

into the muscle for recording motor unit activity. In these disorders, a single stimulus produces prolonged depolarization of the postsynaptic membrane. In the case of acetylcholinesterase deficiency, it is due to failure of breakdown of acetylcholine and resultant sustained activation of postsynaptic receptors. In slow-channel syndrome, the sustained depolarization is due to prolonged open time of the ion channel associated with the acetylcholine receptor.

Routine NCV and EMG is performed in all patients to look for neuropathies or myopathies that could be confused with genetic myasthenia. Transitory neonatal myasthenia occurs in children of myasthenic mothers. Repetitive stimulation at 3 Hz produces a decremental response.

Botulism

Botulism is due to toxins isolated from one of several strains of Clostridium botulinum. Types A, B, and E are responsible for most poisonings in humans. Botulinum toxin (BTX) interferes with release of acetylcholine from the presynaptic terminal. Miniature end-plate potential amplitude is usually normal, but the frequency is very low. End-plate potential amplitude is reduced.

Nerve-conduction studies are normal except for reduced compound motor action potential (CMAP) amplitude. Successive stimuli result in a further reduction in CMAP amplitude. The EMG shows small MUPs initially because of a reduced number of functioning neuromuscular junctions. Later, signs of acute denervation develop. Repetitive stimulation at slow rates produces a decremental response. Repetitive stimulation at fast rates produces a small initial decrement followed by a much more pronounced increment.

The diagnosis of botulism depends on the response to paired stimuli. At short interstimulus intervals (less than 15 ms) the response to the second pulse is greater than to that of the first. This is because the second impulse activates some terminals that were not activated by the first pulse, due to summation of end-plate potentials.

Myasthenic Syndrome

Myasthenic (Eaton-Lambert) syndrome is characterized by progressive weakness without sensory loss, often in association with systemic malignancy. The etiology of the weakness is not completely known, but is felt to be due to circulating factors that interfere with release of transmitter from the presynaptic terminal. The effect is similar to that of botulism, where a bacterial toxin inhibits transmitter release.

The NCVs are normal except for marked reduction in CMAP amplitude. Repetitive stimulation at 3 Hz depresses the CMAP further, giving a marked decremental response. Repetitive stimulation at low rates produces a decremental response. Repetitive stimulation at high rates produces an incremental response, similar to that of botulism. Sensory conduction studies are normal. The EMG shows repetitive discharge of single motor units, due to incremental activation.

Paired stimulation at short interstimulus intervals results in facilitation of the second response. This is similar to the response seen in botulism. However, in contrast, paired stimuli with interstimulus intervals of greater than 15 ms also results in facilitation of the second response. The pathophysiology of the facilitation with short and long latency paired stimuli is different. Therefore, this represents an actual facilitation of transmitter release.

27

□ □ □
□ □ □
□ □ □

Troubleshooting in Nerve-Conduction Studies and Electromyography

Common Pitfalls of Nerve-Conduction Studies and Electromyography

Common Errors Encountered in Nerve-Conduction Studies

Early Positive Component to the Compound Motor Action Potential

A propagating action potential should produce a negative deflection in a surface electrode as it passes. The appearance of an initial small positive potential is usually caused by poor positioning of the surface electrodes. Either the active electrode is not centered over the end-plate zone, or the reference electrode is positioned over an excited membrane. These conditions can be corrected by placing the recording electrode squarely over the muscle belly, and placing the reference distally on an area of skin overlying bone.

Unstable Waveform of the Compound Motor Action Potential or Sensory Neural Action Potential

Unstable waveform is usually due to poor fixation of the recording electrodes. Movement of the limb with stimulation dislodges the electrodes and changes the recording geometry. New gel should be used and the electrodes firmly reapplied.

No Recordable Potentials

A completely flat baseline is not normal. Baseline activity should be present even if the nerve is completely degenerated. Tap the recording electrodes to produce artifact. If this does not produce a response, check that the electrode junction box is switched on, cables are firmly in their sockets, and the gain properly set. If this fails, look further to determine if an electrode lead is broken. This is best accomplished by using a completely different electrode set.

In most machines, a disconnected electrode results in high-amplitude 60-Hz artifact. However, some amplifiers block in response to high-amplitude potentials, that is, they transiently fail to amplify anything, and then gradually recover. During the recovery phase, the baseline activity slowly increases in amplitude.

Excessive 60-Hertz Interference

Excessive 60-Hz interference is usually due to one of the following problems: (1) poor grounding, (2) unequal electrode impedances, or (3) high-amplitude electronic noise in the vicinity. Poor grounding occurs if the ground electrode is old and has breaks in some strands of wire, if the ground electrode was moved several times during the study without replenishing gel or tape, or if the ground electrode has poor electrical continuity with the skin. Some electrode boxes have two sockets for ground, in order to accommodate different size plugs. Only one should be used; using both augments 60-Hz interference.

Unequal electrode impedances can degrade common mode rejection, causing increased 60-Hz artifact. High-amplitude electronic noise is prominent when there are power trunk lines or high-power equipment in the vicinity. Our laboratory has had special difficulty with interference from centrifuges, fluorescent lights, oscilloscopes, and computers.

An occasional cause of augmented 60-Hz interference is excessive length of electrode leads. Stray capacitance and inductance create noise that is dependent on the length of the electrode leads. This is more apt to be a problem during portable studies rather than during studies in the electromyography (EMG) laboratory. The noise can be minimized by keeping the leads short but lengthening the cable from the electrode box.

Mistaking F Wave for H Reflex

Mistaking F wave for H reflex is a common error. While performing an H reflex, it is important to assure that the reflex appears before the direct compound motor action potential (CMAP) as the stimulus intensity is increased, and that the reflex response disappears with maximal stimulation of the nerve. At maximal stimulation an F wave usually occurs at about the same latency as the H reflex response.

High-Voltage Long-Duration Stimulus Required for Stable Wave

A high-voltage long-duration stimulus is usually due to improper positioning of the stimulating electrode. If the probe is not positioned immediately overlying the nerve, more charge is required to depolarize the distant axons. When high-voltage stimuli are used, the nerve may be activated a considerable distance from the probe and the measures of distance are no longer accurate.

Common Errors Encountered in Electromyography

No recordable potentials and 60-Hz interference are encountered in EMG studies as well. The solutions are the same. A few potentials errors are unique to EMG.

Poor Motor Unit Potential Waveform

The normal morphology of motor unit potentials (MUPs) is degraded if the electrode is distant from the active muscle fibers, especially when the electrodes are inserted into superficial fascia. The electrode should be repositioned if the MUPs do not meet the criteria described in chapter 21, "Electromyography." Also, be sure that the patient is making the required contraction. If the patient does not perform the task correctly, the muscle being studied may not be activated, even though the electrode is properly positioned. The distant motor unit potentials are from nearby muscles. If monopolar electrodes are used, poor MUP waveform can be helped by moving the surface reference closer to the needle electrode.

Fibrillation Potentials with Poor Motor Unit Potential Waveform

If the electrode is outside the muscle, MUPs will have poor waveform, and fibrillation potentials will not be seen. However, insertion of the needle into a tendon may result in spontaneous discharges, which look like fibrillations, generated at the myotendinous junction. The morphology of the motor units is degraded. The needle should be repositioned.

Ultra-Short Duration Spontaneous Potentials

Ultra-short duration spontaneous potentials can resemble fibrillation potentials but are of much shorter duration. They tend to follow the electrode; that is, movement of the electrode often does not abolish the activity. This is the EMG equivalent of the electrode pop seen on electroencephalography (EEG).

Mistaking Voluntary Activity for Spontaneous Activity

Voluntary activity may seem to be spontaneous activity in patients who cannot relax. This is especially true in the elderly. Distant motor unit activity can be mistaken for positive sharp waves. Avoid this problem by only interpreting potentials that have a fast upstroke.

Mistaking Phasic Activation for Polyphasic Potentials

Phasic activation can be mistaken for polyphasic potentials if there is excessive reliance on audio output rather than on visual analysis. During phasic muscle activation, multiple motor units may discharge almost simultaneously. The sound is raspy and suggests a polyphasic potential. Reproducible polyphasic potentials are not present on visual inspection. Phasic activation is most common in elderly individuals and in patients with upper motoneuron disorders.

Mistaking Complex Repetitive Discharge for Myotonia

Close analysis of the onset and offset of the discharge and of the change in frequency during the discharge should clearly distinguish complex repetitive discharges from myotonia.

Common Errors in Repetitive Stimulation

The most common reason for a false positive decremental response is poor fixation of the stimulating and recording electrodes, which is especially prominent with testing of proximal muscles. The distance of the electrode from the nerve can be increased by contraction of surrounding muscle.

The most common error in repetitive stimulation is interpretation. A decremental response is supportive of myasthenia gravis, but can also be seen in other disorders, especially with denervation.

Anatomic Variation

The most common anatomic anomalies are the Martin-Gruber anomaly and the accessory peroneal nerve.

Martin-Gruber Anomaly

The Martin-Gruber anastomosis is a connection between the median and ulnar nerves (Figure 27.1). Fibers from the median nerve cross to the ulnar nerve in the forearm. The median fibers innervate any of several muscles that are normally ulnar-innervated. These include the abductor digiti minimi, adductor pollicis, and first dorsal interosseus. The innervation may be derived from both the median and ulnar nerves.

Conduction studies produce a CMAP that is larger after stimulation of the median nerve at the elbow than at the wrist. This is because stimulation at the wrist does not activate the thenar muscles innervated by the anomalous median nerve axons.

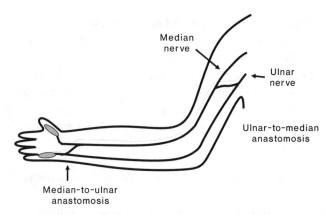

Figure 27.1   Martin-Gruber anomaly. Axons from the ulnar nerve cross over to the median nerve in the arm. Distally in the forearm, they cross again to the ulnar nerve.

The collision technique can be used to diagnose this anomaly. Refer to Figure 27.1 during this discussion. A CMAP is recorded in response to stimulation of the median nerve at the wrist. Then, the stimulus is delivered to the median nerve at the elbow. Third, the stimulus is delivered to the ulnar nerve at the wrist. Fourth, stimuli are delivered to both the median nerve at the elbow and ulnar nerve at the wrist. The action potential from ulnar stimulation propagates antidromically until it collides with the orthodromic action potentials of nerves destined for the ulnar nerve. The action potentials in those nerves will not reach the hand.

Variations in Innervation of Hand Muscles

There are several potential variations in innervation of the intrinsic muscles of the hand, often involving the flexor pollicis brevis or adductor pollicis. These muscles may be innervated exclusively by the median nerve, exclusively by the ulnar nerve, or by both.

Accessory Peroneal Nerve

The common peroneal nerve bifurcates into the deep and superficial peroneal nerves. The deep peroneal innervates the tibialis anterior and extensor digitorum brevis (EDB). In approximately 25% of patients, a branch of the superficial peroneal extends behind the lateral malleolus and turns to innervate the lateral aspect of the EDB. The clue to presence of an accessory peroneal nerve is that the CMAP with stimulation at the knee is larger than with stimulation near the ankle. An accessory peroneal nerve should be mentioned in the comment section of the report, but should be interpreted as normal.

Pathological States

Patients with polyneuropathies may have superimposed mononeuropathies that are clinically significant. Some clinical neurophysiologists believe that in the setting of polyneuropathy, mononeuropathies should not be diagnosed; however, patients may benefit from treatment of the mononeuropathy. Should a patient with diabetic neuropathy not be treated for his carpal tunnel syndrome?

There are no firm guidelines on what constitutes significant slowing of conduction when generalized neuropathic changes are seen. Our laboratory uses 10 meters per second (10 m/sec) discrepancy in conduction velocity. This is reasonable for most studies. However, patients with peripheral neuropathies may have sufficient slowing of distal segments such that conduction across the elbow may not be slowed by 10 m/sec. Our laboratory does not interpret focal slowing unless it is at least 10 m/sec but in the presence of a polyneuropathy the impression might read: "Abnormal study consistent with a peripheral polyneuropathy. Conduction in motor axons across the elbow was slowed in comparison to distal conduction, but the difference was less than 10 m/sec. Focal compression of the ulnar nerve at the elbow is possible but cannot be diagnosed by this study."

If the EMG portion of the study shows clear-cut denervation in an ulnar distribution, the impression can be stronger. A ulnar neuropathy can be diagnosed, but mention should be made of the peripheral polyneuropathy.

Evoked Potentials

28

Electrophysiological Basis of Evoked Potentials

Sensory evoked potentials are the responses of nervous tissue to stimulation. Motor evoked potentials are the responses of muscles to stimulation of the motor cortex. Motor evoked potentials are not commonly used in routine clinical practice, so their discussion will be limited (chapter 33). Most of this section will concentrate on sensory evoked potentials. The three clinically useful modalities of sensory stimulation are auditory, visual, and somatosensory.

The important role of sensory evoked potentials in the diagnosis of multiple sclerosis, transverse myelitis, optic neuritis, acoustic neuromas, and other disorders has been modified by the development of magnetic resonance imaging (MRI). However, sensory evoked potential technology continues to serve an important function in the evaluation of optic neuropathy and myelopathy, in screening for acoustic neuroma, and in intraoperative monitoring of central nervous system function. Somatosensory evoked potentials (SEP) are used to monitor both spinal-cord function during corrective surgery for scoliosis and cerebral function during carotid surgery. Brainstem auditory evoked potentials (BAEPs) are used to monitor some posterior fossa explorations. It is likely that intraoperative monitoring will be the predominant future role of sensory evoked potentials.

Evoked potentials (EPs) are very low amplitude responses superimposed on normal electroencephalographic activity. The responses to many trials must be averaged to make the potentials stand out from background activity. The visual evoked potential (VEP) is the only one that is seen without averaging. It can be observed on routine electroencephalograms (EEG) during low-frequency photic stimulation.

Neural Generators of Evoked Potentials

There are many generators of EPs, since responses are recorded from multiple sites along the afferent pathways. The VEP is most likely due to charge movement associated with conduction in the projections from the lateral geniculate to the visual cortex. Any SEP activity is due to thalamocortical projections, but impulses conducted in peripheral nerves and the dorsal columns are recorded as well. The BAEP is recorded from the nerve volley in the eighth cranial nerve and potentials generated by tracts and nuclei in the brainstem. Specific locations of generators are discussed in the individual sections on VEP, BAEP, and SEP.

The generators of EPs are of two basic types: nerve-fiber bundles and nuclei. Nerve-fiber bundles include both peripheral nerves and central tracts. The recorded potential is due to the advancing front of the compound action potential. The vector of this potential is determined by the direction of projection of the axons.

Potentials generated in nuclei are not easily described by vectors and axonal conduction. Movement of charge in nuclei is a combination of axonal action potentials and charge movement during synaptic transmission. Synapses are oriented in virtually all directions on a cell's dendrites and soma, such that it is impossible to predict the ultimate vector of positivity and negativity. Also, because of the complex orientation of the synapses, there is no guarantee that the field will conform to a simple dipole. Therefore, hypotheses of the sources of individual EP waves are developed on the basis of human pathology and animal studies in addition to a knowledge of basic neuroanatomy.

Theory of Averaging

The EPs are of very small amplitude, and in most instances cannot be seen without averaging. The EP is superimposed on higher-amplitude EEG activity unrelated to the stimulus, and other potentials, such as movement artifact and EMG. Averaging brings out the EP by the assumption that most potentials not caused by the stimulus occur in a random fashion, and will not produce a potential of substantial amplitude after averaging many trials. This assumption is generally true but has two possible sources of error. First, the stimulus may cause a slight movement of the patient that is sufficiently reproducible from trial-to-trial to be detectable in the average. An experienced neurophysiologist can usually identify such abnormal waveforms. Second, 60-Hz interference can appear to be a high-amplitude sinusoidal wave on averaging. To prevent this latter error, the stimulus rate should not be an even harmonic of 60 Hz. The electronics of averaging and analog-to-digital conversion is discussed in detail in part I, "Basic Electronics."

Artifact Rejection

Artifact rejection is an important part of noise reduction. An electronic window is created within specified times and voltages. Potentials larger than the set voltage window are rejected from the average. If a trial contains a potential outside of the window, the entire trial is considered unreliable, and therefore is rejected. When a trial is rejected, an indicator usually shows this on the screen. Also, at the end of the averaging period, most EP machines will display the percent of trials that were rejected.

The time window serves several purposes. Acquisition of data is delayed by a short interval, in part to prevent stimulus artifact from affecting the input amplifier. This is most important for SEPs; however, there can be an element of stimulus artifact with BAEPs due to current movement in the earphone leads. Pattern reversal VEPs have virtually no stimulus artifact. Limiting the duration of recording is important for resolution of the waves, since for averaging each point must be converted into digital format. The number of points that can be remembered is limited by computer memory and governed by the number of channels being recorded, the total time to be sampled, and the time between samples. See part I for details. The following formula shows this relationship:

$$\text{Number of Samples} = \frac{\text{Channels} \times \text{Duration}}{\text{Sample interval}}$$

where *channels* is the number of channels being recorded, *duration* is the time being averaged, and *sample interval* is the time between samples. For most EPs, at least 256 and preferably 512 samples per trial are needed. If four channels are recorded, there are 2,048 samples for each run, and if two trials are recorded, 4,096 data points must be stored in memory. While an EP machine remembers only the running averages, not each trial, available memory can be quickly depleted by recording several averages of several channels each.

29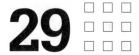

General Principles of Evoked Potentials

This section discusses the general principles of performance and interpretation of evoked potentials (EPs). Much of this also applies to other neurodiagnostic tests but is specifically directed toward the applications of EPs.

The three major modalities of EPs will be discussed individually later in this section. The recommended parameters for stimulation and recording are derived in part from the *Guidelines* (American Electroencephalographic Society 1986).

Evoked Potential Equipment

The equipment used to record EPs is similar to that used for routine EEG and EMG studies and should fulfill the guidelines for electrical safety outlined in part I, "Basic Electronics." In general, modern and well-maintained machines meet the required limitations on allowable leakage current. However, unsafe practices can endanger a patient even with the best equipment. The greatest risk is with somatosensory evoked potentials (SEPs), since the stimulus is an electrical pulse. The patient must be adequately grounded so that the path of current cannot traverse the heart or spinal cord. Normally, the path of current is between the two electrodes of the stimulator; however, current can flow from stimulating electrode to ground if one lead has poor skin contact or high impedance.

Calibration

Evoked potential equipment should be calibrated before each recording session by recording and averaging electronically generated calibration pulses. This procedure assures that there is no problem with data acquisition and manipulation.

The calibration pulses may have one of two sources. Most EP machines have calibration outputs, that is, the output of a signal generator of defined frequency and amplitude. Such waveform generators are technically much simpler than the amplifiers and A/D converters that make up the essentials of the EP machine, so failure of the calibration pulse generator is very unusual. Alternatively, external calibration pulse generators are available at low cost. When triggered by the stimulator, these produce potentials of defined amplitude. Realistically, careful amplitude calibration is not as important as time calibration, since latency is a more important measure than amplitude. Amplitude abnormalities do not contribute significantly to clinical interpretation if the waves are readily identifiable.

Replications

Two replications of each waveform are recommended for each EP. Consistency of waveforms is best visualized if the traces are superimposed on the hard copy. Four replications may be necessary when recording SEPs to provide convincing identification of individual waves. This is usually not necessary when recording brainstem auditory evoked potentials (BAEPs) and visual evoked potentials (VEPs), but should be done if the identification is not obvious.

Normative Data

Normative data from Vanderbilt University Hospital Neurodiagnostic Laboratory are presented in the respective sections on BAEP, VEP, and SEP, and are summarized in the bibliography. However, testing equipment and environment differ between laboratories, and each laboratory should establish its own set of normative data. There are significant maturational effects on the latency of EPs, and the *Guidelines* recommends that normative data be established for each week of the perinatal period, for each month of infancy, and for each decade thereafter. At least twenty subjects from each age group should be tested for each evoked response. Responses from the left and right sides of the same subject cannot be treated as two subjects. This data is used to establish normative data on interside differences in latency and amplitude.

Normative data is expressed as mean ± standard deviation. A latency is considered abnormal if it exceeds 2.5 or 3 standard deviations from the mean. Some laboratories use 2 standard deviations; however, this allows an unacceptable percentage of false-positive interpretations. Linear regression analysis allows a more precise evaluation of waveform latencies as a function of increasing age. However, the relationship between age and latency is not strictly linear and such a level of precision is not needed.

Interpretation

When recordings are made from bipolar linkages, up or down is determined by which electrode is considered active, and which is considered the reference. For routine EEG recording, a negative potential delivered to the

---

St. Nowhere's Hospital Neurodiagnostic Laboratory

Name: Doe, John   Number: 12345
Age: 13   Sex: M

Physician: A. Brown
Study: Visual Evoked Potential

Clinical: New onset of decreased vision in the right eye.
Data:

	Left	Right	Interside difference
	97.6	134.0	36.4
	16	12	4

Comment:

The absolute latency of the P100 from stimulation of the right eye is prolonged. The interside difference in P100 latency is prolonged.

Impression:

Abnormal visual evoked potential study, consistent with a lesion in the right optic nerve.

Jim Doe, M.D.

Figure 29.1   Sample visual evoked potential report. Comment section states the abnormalities. Impression section presents the clinical implication of the findings. The VEP traces are shown on a separate sheet.

active electrode is shown as an upward deflection of the pen. Polarity conventions are not firmly established for display of EP waveforms and the *Guidelines* makes no recommendations in this regard. Many laboratories display the waveforms so that the waves of prominent interest are upward. Since waves of differing polarities are of interest, especially in SEPs and VEPs, it seems most logical to represent the polarity of EP and EEG in the same direction, and to use standard montages, which would facilitate comparisons of recordings between laboratories.

Reports should be concise but thorough. A sample report is shown in Figure 29.1. It is most helpful to put the data in tabular form. Highlighting abnormal values is also helpful. The interpretation can have two sections. The first describes what is abnormal, and the second gives the implications of the abnormalities. Interpretation of the data in light of the clinical history is essential, since many physicians ordering EPs are not experts in this field.

Hard copies of the waveforms should be kept with the patient's record in the laboratory. Some equipment allows for selected waves to be printed on the report along with the tabular data. This is helpful for other neurophysiologists, but not of interest to most clinicians.

30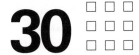

Brainstem Auditory Evoked Potential

The brainstem auditory evoked potential (BAEP) is the complex of potentials produced by the brain and acoustic nerve in response to auditory stimulation. Most of the waves originate in the brainstem. The main use of BAEPs is for evaluation of patients with reduced hearing or with suspected disorders of the brainstem. A particularly sensitive and inexpensive method to screen for acoustic neuromas, BAEPs are also used for intraoperative monitoring during surgery for posterior fossa lesions. The BAEP has less utility for demyelinating disease than visual evoked potentials (VEPs) and somatosensory evoked potentials (SEPs).

Stimulus

Headphones are placed on the subject for delivery of the auditory stimulus. For older children and adults, the headphones are similar to those used for conventional stereo equipment. They completely envelope the ear, thereby reducing ambient noise. For infants and younger children, special earphones are placed into the external auditory canal because regular headphones can collapse the external canals of infants. Both sets of headphones should be provided with evoked potential (EP) machines.

The EP apparatus delivers electronic signals to the headphones, producing movement of the diaphragm. Three types of sounds are produced by the phones: clicks, pure tones, and white noise.

Type of Stimulus

Clicks, most commonly used for routine BAEP testing, are produced by a square-wave pulse delivered to the headphone. The rising phase of the pulse moves the diaphragm in one direction and the fall of the pulse returns the diaphragm to its original position. An initial movement of the diaphragm toward the eardrum is termed *condensation* and away from the ear drum is termed *rarefaction*. These terms are derived from the roots *condense*, "to make more dense," and *rarify*, "to make less dense." Evoked potential machines can deliver both types of movement, but rarefaction is predominantly used for interpretation of routine studies.

Pure tones are generated by some but not all EP machines. The stimulator delivers exact frequencies to the headphones. The most common use for this type of stimulus is pure tone audiometry. Pure tones are not used for routine BAEP but are useful for testing hearing at different frequencies. Some disorders, such as the hearing loss associated with ototoxic drugs, produce a predominant high-frequency hearing loss that is less well detected by BAEP using clicks than by pure tone audiometry.

White noise is sound composed of all audible frequencies in equal proportions. It is similar to the "hush" sound made by a radio that is not tuned to an active station. During BAEP testing, a similar sound is delivered into the ear not being stimulated with clicks. This is called *masking*. Without masking, the ear not being tested could be stimulated by bone conduction of the click delivered to the opposite ear. Strictly speaking, white noise is difficult to produce, so a similar sound is generated that does not have all frequencies exactly equally represented (pink noise).

Stimulus Rate

Clicks are delivered at 8 to 10/sec. This allows for reproducible identification of all waves. Waves I, II, VI, and VII are reduced in amplitude at faster frequencies.

Stimulus Intensity

Terminology for stimulus intensity is potentially confusing. The *Guidelines* recommends that intensity be indicated in units of Decibels (dB) Peak Equivalent Sound Pressure Level, or dB pe SPL. This is measured directly by a sound meter using a constant stimulus of the same frequency and amplitude as the test stimulus to be measured. The dB scale is a log scale, so zero dB is defined as a pressure of 20 micropascals. An alternative scale occasionally used is in reference to normal hearing threshold: dB HL (for Hearing Level). Zero dB HL is the threshold for hearing for a population of normal people. This is approximately equivalent to 30 dB pe SPL. Sensation Level (dB SL) is in reference to the ear being tested. Zero dB SL is the threshold for that ear.

The *Guidelines* recommends stimulus intensities between 40 and 120 dB pe SPL. Many EP machines do not give stimuli louder than that recommended. For routine BAEP, intensity is set at approximately 65 dB SL or HL. Reducing stimulus intensity is only necessary if waveform identification is difficult. With decreasing stimulus intensity, waves II and VI are reduced more than the other waves, allowing for more accurate identification of waves I, III, and V.

Electrode Placement and Recording Parameters

Electrodes are placed in the following positions: (1) A1, behind the left ear; (2) A2, behind the right ear; and (3) Cz, at the vertex. These surface electrodes are identical in composition to those used for routine electroencephalography (EEG) recording. Detailed guidelines for placement of surface electrodes are included in part II, "Electroencephalography."

Recommended montages for recording of BAEP are Cz-Ai for channel 1, and Cz-Ac for channel 2, where Cz is at the vertex, Ai is behind the ipsilateral ear, and Ac is behind the contralateral ear. Positions Ai and Ac are identical to A1 and A2 in the 10-20 Electrode Placement System for EEG surface electrode placement, described in part II. Cz is identical to the position Cz in the 10-20 system.

Therefore, for stimulation of each ear, the first channel records the difference in potential between the ipsilateral ear and the vertex, while the second channel records the difference between the contralateral ear and vertex. Recording from the contralateral ear aids in identification of waves I, IV, and V.

Stimulus and recording parameters are summarized in Table 30.1.

Waveform Identification and Origin

The waves routinely analyzed in BAEP are numbered I through V. Waves VI and VII are also identified but not used in interpretation. Waves I and V should be identified first. Wave I is generated by the distal portion of the acoustic nerve and is approximately 2 ms after the stimulus. Wave I identification is aided by recording from a contralateral electrode derivation; it is the only wave present on ipsilateral but not contralateral recording.

Wave V may be generated by projections from the pons to the midbrain. There are several criteria for identifying wave V; it normally appears at approximately 6 ms and is often combined with wave IV into a single complex waveform. Wave V is also the first waveform whose falling edge dips below the baseline.

The IV–V complex has a wider separation with recording from the contralateral ear than recording from the ipsilateral ear. This means that the contralateral wave IV is of slightly shorter latency and wave V is of slightly longer latency. Wave V is the last to disappear as stimulus intensity is decreased.

Wave III is thought to be generated by the projections from the superior olive through the lateral lemniscus. It is the major peak between waves I and V.

Table 30.1 Brainstem Auditory Evoked Potential Stimulus and Recording Parameters

Stimulus Parameters	
Rate	8–10/sec
Intensity	65 dB SL
Number of trials	1,000–4,000
Recommended montages	
Channel 1	Cz–Ai
Channel 2	Cz–Ac
Recording Parameters	
Low-frequency filter	10–30 Hz (–3 dB)
High-frequency filter	2,500–3,000 Hz (–3 dB)
Analysis time	15 ms
Number of trials	1,000–4,000
Measurements	Wave I peak latency
	Wave III peak latency
	Wave V peak latency
	I–III interpeak interval
	III–V interpeak interval
	Wave I amplitude
	Wave V amplitude
	Wave V/I amplitude ratio

Note: Special circumstances may occasionally dictate changes in these standard parameters.

Source: Derived from American Electroencephalographic Society 1986.

The amplitude of wave III is often decreased on contralateral recording.

Waves I, III, and IV are the major peaks used in interpretation. Waves II and IV are between I and III, and III and V, respectively. Their latency and amplitude is variable.

Interpretation of Data

Latency is a more important measure than amplitude in the interpretation of BAEP data. The most important measurements are wave I latency, wave I–III interpeak latency, and wave III–V interpeak latency. A sample normal BAEP is shown in Figure 30.1. Normative data are shown in Table 30.2.

Increased wave I latency is seen if the most distal portion of the acoustic nerve is affected. Most acoustic neuromas do not affect wave I.

Increased I–III interpeak latency indicates a defect in the pathway from the proximal eighth nerve into the inferior pons. The lesion may be either in the nerve or in the brainstem. This is the most common abnormality found in patients with acoustic neuromas (see Figure 30.2).

Increased III–V interpeak latency indicates a defect in conduction between the caudal pons and midbrain (see Figure 30.3). Increased I–III and III–V

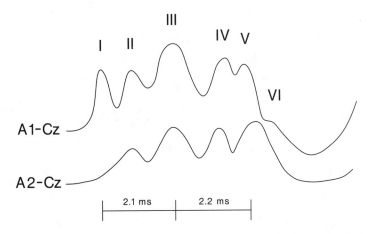

Figure 30.1 Normal brainstem auditory evoked potential. Waves are numbered according to conventions described in the text. The top trace was recorded from the ipsilateral side, while the bottom trace was recorded from the contralateral side.

interpeak latencies indicate that the lesion is affecting both the brainstem above the caudal pons and either the caudal pons or the acoustic nerve. In most instances, the prominent lesion is in the pons.

Absence of wave I with normal III and V may indicate a peripheral hearing disorder, with the caveat that conduction in the caudal pons cannot be evaluated. Absence of wave I with prolonged latency or absence of waves III and/or V usually indicates a defect of conduction in the eighth nerve along with a lesion in the caudal pons; however, this is difficult to evaluate without a recordable I–III interpeak interval.

Absence of wave III with normal waves I and V is normal but if the I–V interval is prolonged, then a lesion affecting conduction somewhere from the eighth nerve to the midbrain is suspected.

Table 30.2 Brainstem Auditory Evoked Potential Normal Data

Waveform	Male	Female
Wave I latency	2.10	2.10
I–III interpeak interval	2.55	2.40
III–V interpeak interval	2.35	2.20
I–V interpeak interval	4.60	4.45
Interside I–V difference	0.50	0.50
V/I amplitude ratio	0.50	0.50

Note: All latencies are given in milliseconds (ms) and represent the upper limit of normal. The V/I amplitude ratio is a simple ratio, without units. These data are used at Vanderbilt University Hospital.

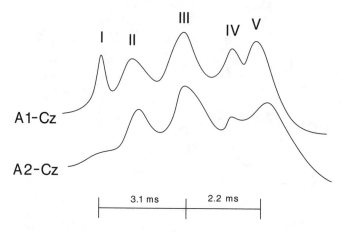

Figure 30.2   Increased I–III interpeak interval of the BAEP. This is due to a lesion between the intracranial portion of the eighth nerve and caudal pons.

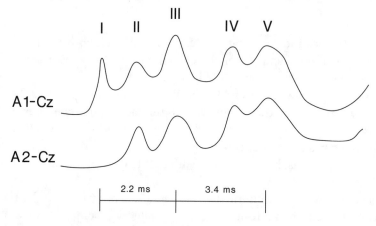

Figure 30.3   Increased III–V interpeak interval of the BAEP. This is due to a lesion above the caudal pons.

Absence of wave V with normal waves I and III is uncommon, but when present it indicates a lesion affecting the auditory pathways above the caudal pons. This is considered an extreme prolongation of the III–V interval.

Pediatric Brainstem Auditory Evoked Potentials

Brainstem Auditory Evoked Potentials for Disorders of Childhood

Often, BAEPs are used to evaluate children with suspected hearing loss, especially infants and children who cannot cooperate with conventional audiometry. An abnormal BAEP is usually associated with abnormalities on behavioral testing of hearing; however, a normal BAEP does not guarantee normal hearing. If the lesion is of the peripheral auditory structures, threshold may be increased, but there may not be a change in I–V interpeak interval.

Abnormal BAEPs are recorded in children with several metabolic disorders: phenylketonuria, maple syrup urine disease, nonketotic hyperglycinemia, and Leigh's disease. Wave I–V interpeak interval is typically increased. However, the BAEP is not important in the diagnosis of these disorders, since the abnormalities are not disease-specific.

Neonatal BAEP

Special care is needed in recording BAEPs in the newborn. Ordinary headphones may produce sufficient pressure to close off the external auditory canal. The result is absent or poor waveforms. Special earphones that do not deform the canal are routinely provided with EP machines.

Sedation is usually required to record EPs in neonates. This is best accomplished by the use of chloral hydrate, meperidine plus secobarbital, or meperidine plus promethazine plus chlorpromazine (DPT). Sedation does not affect short-latency EPs, such as the BAEP.

The BAEP is performed in an infant for evaluation of respiratory and feeding dysfunction, particularly with suspected perinatal asphyxia and in prematures. The I–V interpeak latency is prolonged in prematures, and may be related to delayed maturity of brainstem nuclei and pathways. There is an almost linear relationship between the decline in I–V interpeak latency and the reduction in apnea frequency.

The I–V interpeak interval is increased in term newborns who have experienced episodes of total asphyxia with subsequent damage to brainstem nuclei. The mortality and neurologic morbidity in such newborns is high. Newborns who have experienced prolonged partial asphyxia sustain mainly hemispheric damage and the I–V interval may be normal despite a poor neurologic outcome.

Brainstem Auditory Evoked Potential in Specific Disorders

Acoustic Neuromas

Prolongation of the I–III interpeak interval is the most sensitive finding in the diagnosis of acoustic neuroma. If there is difficulty in obtaining wave I, the technician should place an electrode in the external auditory canal for better recording. Alternatively, electrocochleography can aid with identification of wave I. In patients with very large tumors, there may be such severe damage that there are no reproducible waves after I. In very early cases, the BAEP has not been normal when imaging revealed an acoustic neuroma. A sample finding with acoustic neuroma is shown in Figure 30.2.

Brainstem Tumors and Stroke

The BAEP is abnormal in most patients with intrinsic tumors of the brainstem. This is especially true in patients with pontine involvement. The usual abnormality is delay or loss or waves III and V and increased I–III and III–V interpeak intervals.

The BAEP is also abnormal in most patients with brainstem stroke. However, a few patients with extensive brainstem infarctions have been reported to have normal BAEPs. In some of these patients the amplitudes of the waveforms were low; however, amplitude abnormalities are not emphasized in the interpretation of BAEPs. Approximately 50% of patients with transient ischemic attacks affecting the posterior circulation have latency abnormalities, and 50% of patients who recover from definite brainstem strokes have normal BAEPs. A sample recording from a patient with a brainstem lesion is shown in Figure 30.3.

Multiple Sclerosis

The BAEP is less sensitive than VEPs and SEPs for detection of clinically unsuspected lesions in patients being evaluated for multiple sclerosis (MS). The usual abnormalities are reduction in wave V amplitude and increased III–V interpeak latency.

Most abnormalities are asymmetric, affecting the response from only one ear. Caution in the interpretation of amplitude abnormalities is recommended. The BAEP cannot distinguish demyelinating disease from tumors or infarction.

Coma and Brain Death

The President's Commission on Determination of Cerebral Death cited BAEP as a confirmatory test, along with EEG and radionucleotide brain scan. The commission criteria are cited in the bibliography.

The BAEP is consistent with cerebral death if there are no reproducible waves after I. Wave II may be intact in less than 10% of brain-dead patients, reinforcing the hypothesis that wave II is generated by the intracranial portion of the eighth nerve. The presence of wave II is consistent with cerebral death in a patient who otherwise fulfills all other clinical criteria, and has no subsequent waves on the BAEP.

Miscellaneous Disorders

Abnormal interpeak latencies are reported in patients with meningitis, B_{12} deficiency, epilepsy, alcoholism, and diabetes mellitus. The abnor-

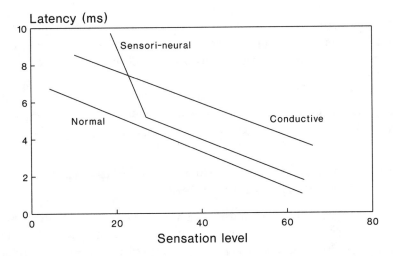

Figure 30.4 Relationship between sensation level and latency of wave V. This is essentially a semilog plot, since sensation level is an exponential parameter. Conductive hearing loss results in an increased latency at all intensities. Sensorineural hearing loss results in recruitment at low intensities but a normal slope at higher intensities.

malities associated with diabetes and meningitis are consistent with a lesion of the acoustic nerve: increased I–III interpeak interval.

Audiometry

Audiometry is a variation of evoked responses that evaluates dysfunction of the ear and proximal eighth nerve. The BAEP technique is the same as described previously, except that special attention is given to the latency of wave V at different stimulus intensities. The wave V latency is plotted against the stimulus intensity at 20, 40, 60, and 80 dB greater than threshold (Figure 30.4). Because of the nature of the decibel scale, this is essentially a semi-log plot.

The relationship between wave V latency and stimulus intensity is linear in normal individuals, with higher intensities producing shorter latencies. Conductive hearing loss does not change the slope of this relationship but does prolong the latency at each intensity. Therefore, the curve is shifted up. The response looks as if the intensities are turned down at every point, which is in effect what occurs with conductive loss. Sensorineural hearing loss produces a curve with two slopes. At low intensities, there is decreased responsiveness of the end-organ, so that for a given intensity the wave V latency is prolonged. With increases in intensity, there is more recruitment of nerves than normal, so that the slope of the curve is steeper. At high intensities, sufficient recruitment has occurred such that the latency may be normal. At this point, the slope reverts to normal. This L-shaped curve is typical for sensorineural hearing loss.

Audiometry is useful for evaluating patients for hearing loss, where the localization of the lesion is in doubt. We also use audiometry to follow patients receiving chemotherapeutic agents that cause ototoxicity.

Intraoperative Monitoring of Brainstem Auditory Evoked Potential

The BAEP is often used as a monitor of brainstem integrity during posterior fossa surgery. It is recorded at intervals, and compared not only to the previous intraoperative recordings, but also to a recording made prior to surgery. Anesthesia has virtually no effect on the BAEP, so that reproducible waveforms are easily recorded in most patients. Monitoring of BAEP is not useful during surgery for acoustic neuroma, since most patients are left with total loss of hearing in the affected ear.

There is concern over incipient damage to the brainstem if there is:

- Loss of normal waveforms after wave I, or
- Decrease in amplitude of a major wave (III, V), or
- Increase interpeak interval (I–III or III–V).

If all of the waves are lost including wave I, there could be failure to generate the click in the earphone, or other technical factors, and caution must be exercised before suggesting brainstem dysfunction. If wave I (and usually also II) is present, with the loss of later waves, this indicates severe abnormality in conduction in auditory pathways through the brainstem. Deterioration of the BAEP after surgery correlates with poor auditory function.

31

Visual Evoked Potential

The visual evoked potential (VEP) is the potential recorded from the occipital region in response to visual stimuli. The stimulus may be presented in several ways (see the next section below). The VEP differs from other evoked responses in that the response is a long-latency response; the brainstem auditory evoked potentials (BAEP) and somatosensory evoked potentials (SEP) are short-latency responses. There are long-latency components to the BAEP and SEP but these are not routinely used for interpretation because they are too variable for clinical usefulness.

The VEP is the only evoked response that is visible without averaging. During routine electroencephalography (EEG), photic stimulation is used to activate epileptiform discharges in patients suspected of having seizures. The photic stimulation is a bright flash delivered to subjects with their eyes closed. At flash frequencies below 5 to 7/sec, an evoked response is recorded from the occipital leads. A driving response is recorded at faster flash frequencies. The VEP is highly reproducible, as long as the patient maintains fixation and has no change in visual acuity.

Stimulus

The VEP stimulus may be flash, full-field pattern reversal, or hemifield pattern reversal. Flash is used in patients who cannot cooperate with the level of fixation required for pattern-reversal stimulation. The latencies of flash stimulation are more variable than pattern-reversal stimulation, so that the flash VEP is only useful to test continuity of the visual pathways. Full-field pattern reversal is the usual stimulus for the VEP. Since each eye is examined separately, this tests the anterior visual pathways especially well. Hemifield pattern-reversal stimulation is used for localization of lesions behind the optic chiasm. While many laboratories still perform hemifield testing, modern imaging procedures have replaced this technique in most laboratories.

Flash Stimulus

The flash stimulus is delivered by a strobe light placed in front of the patient. The device is similar to that used for photic stimulation during routine EEG. Typically, the eyes are closed. Sufficient light passes through the lids to activate the retina.

An intact flash VEP indicates continuity of the pathways from the retina to the lateral geniculate; flash VEPs have been recorded in the absence of a functioning cortex. Therefore, flash stimuli are not used if reproducible waveforms can be obtained with pattern-reversal stimuli.

Pattern-Reversal Stimulus

Pattern-reversal stimulation is generated by a video display attached to a pattern generator or video card connected to a computer. The patient, in a sitting position, fixates on a small target in the middle of the display. On the display is a checkerboard pattern (see Figure 31.1). At regular intervals, the pattern is electronically reversed so that the white squares become black and the black squares become white; thus, there is pattern reversal. The response is recorded from occipital leads and averaged over many trials.

Several parameters influence the response:

- Size of the checks
- Size of the visual field stimulated
- Frequency of pattern reversal

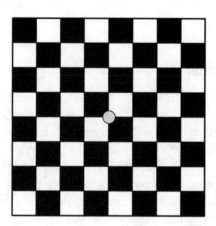

Figure 31.1   Pattern-reversal stimulus for the visual evoked potential. The black-and-white checkerboard pattern is generated on a cathode-ray tube or light-emitting diode array. The black squares become white and the white become black at a rate of twice per second.

Table 31.1 Visual Evoked Potental Stimulus and Recording Parameters

Stimulus Parameters	
Reversal rate	2/sec (500 ms interval)
Contrast	>50%
Check size	28–32 min of arc
Field size	8° of arc
Number of trials	100–200
Recommended electrodes	
Midline occipital (MO)	5 cm above inion
Right occipital (RO)	5 cm right of MO electrode
Left occipital (LO)	5 cm left of MO electrode
Midline frontal (MF)	12 cm above the nasion
Recommended montages	
Channel 1	RO–MF
Channel 2	MO–MF
Channel 3	LO–MF
Recording Parameters	
Low-frequency filter	0.2–1.0 Hz (–3 dB)
High-frequency filter	200–300 Hz (–3 dB)
Analysis time	250 ms
Measurements	N75 latency from each eye
	P100 latency from each eye
	Interocular latency difference
	Amplitude (baseline to P100 or N75 to P100)
	Interocular amplitude ratio (larger/smaller)

Note: Special circumstances may occasionally dictate changes in these standard parameters.

Source: Derived from American Electroencephalographic Society 1986.

- Luminance of the display
- Contrast between background and foreground
- Fixation of the patient.

Table 31.1 summarizes the stimulus and recording parameters for the VEPs.

Check size affects the amplitude and latency of the VEP. Size is measured in minutes of visual field arc, where there are 60 minutes (60') per degree of arc. The maximal response is elicited by a check size between 15' and 60'. The wide range of check size is made possible by differences in other variables, notably size of the stimulus field. With smaller checks the latency of the response is increased and the amplitude is reduced. With larger field sizes the amplitude is reduced. The fovea is stimulated better by smaller checks, and the periphery is stimulated better by larger checks. The recommended check size is 28' to 32' of the visual field arc; this is a compromise between the two extremes.

Stimulus field size should be at least 8 degrees (8°) of the visual field arc, since approximately 80% of the response is generated by the central 8° of vision.

A smaller field size has been recommended to increase sensitivity to subtle defects but the false positive rate is unacceptable. Visual acuity is the limiting factor in the presence of reduced stimulus field and reduced check size.

Reversal rate should be 2/sec, at intervals of 500 ms. Faster reversal rates cause an increase in the latency of the major wave, P100. Rates faster than 5 to 7/sec produce the entrained driving response seen on routine EEG during photic stimulation.

Luminance is not directly mentioned in the *Guidelines*. However, low luminance is known to cause an increase in P100 latency and a decrease in amplitude. Standard video monitors used for routine VEP testing produce sufficient luminance, but this should be checked periodically. Note that pupillary diameter can greatly affect retinal illumination, so marked interside differences in pupil diameter must be considered in interpretation of the VEP.

Contrast between the light and dark squares must be greater than 50%. In practice, the contrast is much greater than this. Lower contrast results in a delayed and lower amplitude P100.

Fixation on the target is helpful, but not essential, for a good reproducible response. Intentional nonfixation does not affect the P100 latencies in most individuals but can cause a reduction of amplitude. Some individuals may be able to voluntarily reduce the amplitude sufficiently to make the P100 not identifiable.

Hemifield Pattern Reversal

Whole-field pattern-reversal stimulation is given to one eye at a time, to test the optic nerve. Hemifield stimulation is given to both eyes simultaneously, but to only one hemifield, either right or left. The pattern-reversal technique is the same as that used for full-field stimulation, with the checkerboard on one side of the screen blocked out. Comparing the responses to stimulation of the two hemifields tests the visual pathways behind the optic chiasm.

Magnetic resonance imaging (MRI) and computerized tomography (CT) provide excellent visualization of the retrochiasmatic visual pathways and are superior to VEP for detection of lesions in these regions. Therefore, we do not commonly use hemifield stimulation for evaluation of patients with suspected brain pathology.

Electrode Placement and Recording Parameters

In most laboratories, electrodes are placed according to the 10-20 Electrode Placement System. Most interpretations are made on the basis of recordings made in the Cz-Oz derivation. Other channels recorded are Oz, Pz, and Cz in reference to either an ear or a noncephalic electrode. While there are significant variations between laboratories, the *Guidelines* recommends that the following electrodes be placed:

MO Midline occipital
RO 5 cm right of MO
LO 5 cm left of MO
MF Midline frontal

The recommendations are outlined in Table 31.1. Recommended montages are:

RO–MF
MO–MF
LO–MF

The laterally placed electrodes facilitate accurate waveform identification, especially for hemifield stimulation. For routine pattern-reversal stimulation, placement of electrodes is dictated by findings. If the waveforms are poor or unusual, use of lateral and/or more anterior electrodes is recommended to look for an unusual potential distribution.

Waveform Identification

Normal Waveforms

Inspection of the normal VEP reveals three identifiable waveforms: N75, P100, and N145 (Figure 31.2). The positive potential at approximately 100 ms (P100) is used for interpretation. The negative N75 and N145 that precede and follow the P100 are helpful for identification but not for routine interpretation.

Variant Waveforms

There are two common variations in the VEP waveform: bifid, and inverted (Figure 31.2). Both are due to variation in the anatomical orientation of the visual cortex and optic radiations. The main clinical concern regarding the bifid pattern is where to call the P100. If the split in the P100 is fairly narrow, it is reasonable to use a point that is extrapolated from the ascending and descending slopes. If the derived P100 latency is normal, then the VEP is interpreted as normal. Some patients will exhibit a widely split P100, not amenable to extrapolation. This may be due to defects in the projection to the upper and lower segments of the calcarine cortex, possibly from visual field defects. Stimulation of only the lower half of the visual field may improve the bifid waveform, but the latency is often abnormal anyway. There is controversy as to whether or not a bifid waveform should be considered abnor-

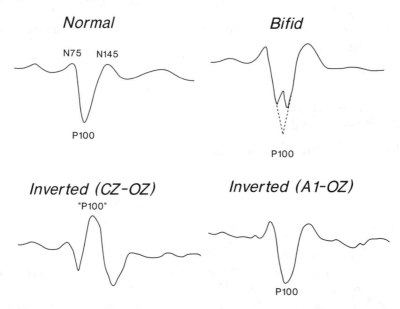

Figure 31.2   Normal visual evoked potentials. The top left wave is the most common observed. The other waveforms are variants of normal, as described in the text.

mal on its own. The most conservative approach is to simplify the waveform by lower half stimulation and localize the P100 by recording from Pz and Cz in addition to Oz; using these techniques, the test is abnormal if the latency of the resultant waveform is increased.

The inverted waveform is an artifact of the montage commonly used in recording the VEP. In some patients, the positivity of the VEP is shifted superiorly and anteriorly. Using a Cz-Oz montage, the Cz electrode is more positive than the Oz electrode, causing a reversed direction of the deflection. N75 and N145 are reversed as well, and one of these could be misinterpreted as the P100. If the waveform is not typical of the normal VEP, recordings should be made from channels other than Cz-Oz, such as A1-Oz, A1-Pz, and A1-Cz. These will allow for mapping of the topography of the VEP, and aid greatly in the identification of the P100.

Interpretation of Data

The best indication for VEP is a suspected disorder of the anterior visual pathways. Disorders of the optic tracts and radiations are better assessed by CT and MRI.

The most common abnormality is an increase in the latency of the P100 from one eye. This indicates a lesion in the optic tract anterior to the chiasm.

If the P100 is prolonged from both eyes, one would suspect bilateral optic nerve lesions, but the same recording could be obtained from a lesion in the region of the chiasm, or from extensive retrochiasmal damage. To distinguish between these possibilities, VEP with hemifield stimulation may be helpful. A lesion in the right optic tract will result in a prolonged P100 with stimulation of the left hemifield.

The absolute latency of the P100 is considered prolonged if it exceeds 117 ms. However, interside latency difference is even more sensitive than absolute latency. For example, if the P100 from full-field stimulation of the left eye is 110 ms, and that from stimulation of the right eye is 97 ms, the study would be interpreted as abnormal. The 13-ms interside difference is excessive, even though the absolute latencies are both within normal limits. Normal values are shown in Table 31.2.

Optic Neuritis

Optic neuritis typically increases the latency of the P100 using the pattern-reversal VEP. If the optic neuritis is unilateral, then the increase is purely unilateral. A prolonged latency of the P100 from an asymptomatic eye suggests a previous subclinical episode of optic neuritis. A sample VEP from a patient with optic neuritis is shown in Figure 31.3.

After the acute phase of the optic neuritis, very few VEPs return to normal. Therefore, if a patient is being evaluated for previous optic neuritis, the VEP should be abnormal.

Multiple Sclerosis

Approximately 15% of patients with optic neuritis will later develop other signs of multiple sclerosis (MS). In patients with optic neuritis, SEPs are often performed to look for clinically silent lesions in the spinal cord. Conversely,

Table 31.2   Visual Evoked Potential Normal Data

Pattern-Reversal Visual Evoked Potential	
Latency	117 ms
Inter-eye latency difference	6 ms
Amplitude	3 μV
Inter-eye amplitude difference	5.5 μV
Flash Visual Evoked Potential	
Latency	132 ms
Inter-eye latency difference	6 ms

Note: Most laboratories do not interpret a study as being abnormal solely on the basis of low or unequal amplitudes. These data are used at Vanderbilt University Hospital.

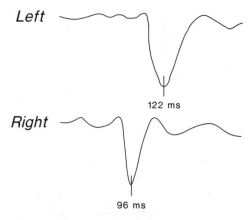

Figure 31.3 Visual evoked potential with left optic neuritis. The response from stimulation of the left eye is prolonged. Upper limit of normal is 117 ms. The response from the right is normal.

when MS is suspected because of lesions in other parts of the central nervous system, VEP may be useful to show previous asymptomatic optic neuritis. Abnormal VEP latency is present in approximately 40% of patients with MS who do not have a history of optic neuritis. Virtually all patients with a history of optic neuritis have either an absolute increase in the latency of the P100 from the affected eye, or an abnormal interside difference in latency, if the absolute latencies are normal.

Tumors

Tumors affecting the anterior visual pathways commonly produce compression of the optic nerve and chiasm. This results in visual field defects that affect each eye differently. The VEP is almost always abnormal, but the correlation between visual acuity and degree of VEP abnormality is poor. Reported abnormalities are alterations in absolute or interside latencies of the P100 and changes in wave morphology and amplitude. Latency changes are more reliable than morphology or amplitude changes.

Tumors affecting the posterior visual pathways are less likely to affect the VEP. Full-field pattern-reversal VEP is usually normal in patients with dense hemianopia. The use of electrodes lateral to Oz may reveal an amplitude asymmetry with the higher amplitude ipsilateral to the side of the lesion, but amplitude asymmetries may be present in normal individuals. Hemifield stimulation reveals abnormalities in some individuals; however, the sensitivity and specificity is not good enough to justify using this technique to screen for posterior lesions. Imaging techniques should be used.

Pseudotumor Cerebri

Patients with pseudotumor cerebri have increased intracranial pressure not associated with a structural defect, such as mass or obstruction in cerebrospinal fluid flow. If the increased pressure is untreated, patients may develop visual loss. If treatment is effective, the visual loss can improve; however, permanent deficits result if there has been long-standing increased pressure.

Most patients with pseudotumor cerebri have normal VEPs. A few patients are described with abnormalities in association with incipient visual loss; however, VEP should not be used as a screening procedure for increased intracranial pressure.

Functional Disorders

The pattern-reversal VEP is frequently used to evaluate patients with suspected functional visual loss. Few individuals can voluntarily suppress the VEP. An intact VEP usually suggests continuity of the visual pathways but does not fully exclude cortical blindness. Caution is needed in using pattern-shift VEP for the diagnosis of functional visual loss.

A normal flash VEP indicates continuity of the visual pathways only to the lateral geniculate. An intact flash response is expected with lesions of the optic radiations and visual cortex. Great care should be exercised in interpretation of latency abnormalities of the flash VEP.

Ocular and Retinal Disorders

Many ocular and retinal disorders cause abnormalities in the pattern-shift VEP. The effect of impaired visual acuity and effective retinal illumination on the VEP were discussed previously. The VEP is not ordinarily used for the diagnosis of these disorders. While some patients with glaucoma have an increased latency and reduced amplitude of the P100, a normal VEP cannot be interpreted as indicating normal intraocular pressure. The effects of ocular and retinal disorders on the VEP is of interest only in the interpretation of VEPs used to evaluate disorders at and behind the optic nerve.

Cortical Blindness

Some patients with documented cortical blindness have normal pattern-reversal VEPs. The use of smaller check size may help to bring out abnormalities; however, this is not routinely done in most neurodiagnostic laboratories.

Intraoperative Monitoring of Visual Evoked Potential

The flash VEP has been used for intraoperative monitoring during surgery in the region of the optic nerve and chiasm with mixed results. An absence of change in VEP waveform or latency is correlated with no postoperative deterioration in vision. The main indications for VEP monitoring are surgery of optic glioma, meningioma in the region of the optic nerve or chiasm, pituitary adenoma, craniopharyngioma, and hypothalamic tumor.

32 □ □ □
□ □ □
□ □ □

Somatosensory Evoked Potential

The somatosensory evoked potential (SEP) is the response to electrical stimulation of peripheral nerves. Stimulation of almost any nerve is possible, but the most commonly studied are median, ulnar, peroneal, and posterior tibial. Recording is made of the afferent nerve volley, the potentials generated in the spinal cord and relay nuclei, and the potentials generated over the motor-sensory cortex. Short-latency responses are used in clinical practice; long-latency responses are too variable to be helpful.

The SEPs are helpful in the diagnosis of spinal-cord disease that is not displayed by imaging studies, especially multiple sclerosis, and are used routinely for intraoperative monitoring of some surgical procedures, such as Harrington rod placement for scoliosis.

Overview of Stimulus and Waveform Generation

The stimulus for SEPs is a brief electric pulse delivered to the distal portion of the nerve. The electrical stimulus cannot selectively activate sensory nerves, so a small muscle twitch is associated. There are no effects of the retrograde volley in motor nerves on central projections of the sensory fibers.

Intensity of the stimulus is adjusted so that there is slight twitching of the innervated muscles. This intensity is sufficient to activate low-threshold myelinated nerve fibers. The compound action potential is conducted through the dorsal roots and into the dorsal columns. The impulses ascend in the dorsal columns to the gracile and cuneate nuclei where the primary afferent fibers synapse on the second order neurons, which ascend through the brainstem to the thalamus. Thalamocortical projections are extensive, as are secondary intracortical associative projections.

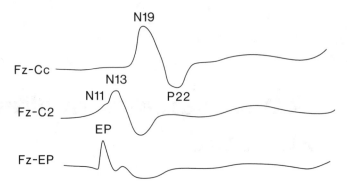

Figure 32.1 Normal median nerve somatosensory evoked potentials. The potentials used for routine analysis are EP, N13, and N19.

Median-Nerve Somatosensory Evoked Potential

Median-nerve SEPs are useful to assess conduction in the upper cervical cord and brain and to assess spinal-cord disease when performed in conjunction with leg SEPs. A delay in conduction from the leg with a normal median response localizes the lesion to the region between the cauda equina and the cervical spinal cord. A sample median SEP is shown in Figure 32.1.

Median Somatosensory Evoked Potential Stimulus and Recording Parameters

A summary of SEP stimulus and recording parameters is presented in Table 32.1. Specific recommendations for median-nerve SEPs are presented in Table 32.2. For median-nerve SEPs, electrodes are placed as follows: (1) Erb's point on each side, (2) over the fifth or second cervical spine process (C5S or C2S), (3) at C3' and C4', and (4) at FZ.

Erb's point is 2 to 3 cm above the clavicle, just lateral to the attachment of the sternocleidomastoid muscle. Stimulation at Erb's point produces abduction of the arm and flexion of the elbow. The second and fifth spinous processes are identified by counting up from the seventh, notable by its prominence at the base of the neck. C3' and C4' are 2-cm posterior to the electrode positions C3 and C4, respectively, of the 10-20 Electrode Placement System. These electrodes are over the motor-sensory cortex. FZ is in the midline-frontal region. This is identical to the FZ electrode position of the 10-20 system used for routine electroencephalography (EEG).

The recommended channels are:

- Contralateral central cortex (C3' or C4'): FZ
- Contralateral central cortex: Erb's point (EP)

Table 32.1   Somatosensory Evoked Potential Stimulus and Recording Parameters

Stimulus Parameters	
Stimulus rate	4–7/sec
Recording Parameters	
Low-frequency filter	5–30 Hz (–3 dB)
High-frequency filter	2,500–4,000 Hz (–3 dB)

Note: See subsequent tables for specific recommendations for individual nerves.

Source: Derived from American Electroencephalographic Society 1986.

Table 32.2   Median Nerve Somatosensory Evoked Potential Stimulus and Recording Parameters

Number of trials	500–2,000
Stimulating electrodes	
Cathode	Median nerve 2 cm proximal to wrist crease
Anode	2 cm distal to cathode
Recording electrodes	2 electrodes at EP
	Cervical spine (C2S or C5S)
	2 cm distal to C3 and C4 (C3' and C4')
	Midline frontal (Fz)
	Behind ears (Ai = ipsilateral and Ac = contralateral)
Montage	
Channel 1	C3' or C4'–Fz or Ac
Channel 2	C3' or C4'–EP contralateral
Channel 3	C5S or C2S–Fz
Channel 4	EP ipsi–EP contra
Measurements	Peak latency of EP potential
	Peak latency of N13 in neck-scalp derivation
	Peak latency of N20 in scalp-scalp or scalp-ear derivation

EP = Erb's point.

Source: American Electroencephalographic Society 1986.

- Neck (C5S or C2S): FZ
- EP ipsilateral: EP contralateral.

The *Guidelines* suggests a recording time of 40 ms, beginning at the onset of the stimulus. Frequently, the first 1 to 5 ms are not recorded to reduce stimulus artifact. Longer recording times should be used only if there are no reproducible potentials. For adequate waveform identification, 500 to 2,000 trials should be averaged.

The recommended filter settings are the same for all of the SEPs: (1) low-frequency filter at 5 to 30 Hz (–3 dB) and high-frequency filter at 2,500 to 4,000

Hz (–3 dB); (2) filter slope not exceeding 12 dB/octave for low frequencies and 24 dB/octave for high frequencies. The *Guidelines* cites an optimal bandpass as 20 to 3,000 Hz. This can be used for all of the following studies.

Median Somatosensory Evoked Potential Waveform Identification

With stimulation of the median nerve, the recorded potentials are from Erb's point, the neck, and the scalp. The potential at Erb's point is termed *EP*; the same potential recorded in the neck-scalp derivation is called *N9*. N11 and N13 are recorded on neck-scalp leads, but only N13 is routinely used for interpretation. N20 and P22 are recorded from the contralateral cortex, but only N20 is used for interpretation. Normative data for all SEPs are presented in Table 32.3.

Median Somatosensory Evoked Potential Interpretation

The median SEP is used for thoracic outlet syndrome, cervical myelopathy, and for intraoperative monitoring during carotid endarterectomy. Increased latency or loss of a waveform during surgery suggests ischemia.

Table 32.3 Somatosensory Evoked Potential Normal Data

Wave	Latency	Interside Difference
Median Nerve SEP		
N9/EP	11.80	0.87
N11	13.90	0.74
N13	16.10	0.06
N20	21.50	1.20
P25	25.60	1.10
N13-N20 interval	7.10	1.20
Peroneal Nerve SEP		
LP	13.50	0.50
P27	31.80	2.24
N33	40.70	5.96
LP-N27 interval	19.38	2.30
Tibial Nerve SEP		
LP	22.10	1.20
P37	41.70	1.40
LP-P37 interval	20.50	1.50

SEP = Somatosensory evoked potential.

Note: All latencies are presented in milliseconds (ms). These data are used at Vanderbilt University Hospital.

Table 32.4   Somatosensory Evoked Potential Waveform Origins

Waveform	Origins
Median	
N9 (EP)	Afferent volley in plexus
N11	Dorsal root entry zone
N13	Dorsal columns and nuclei
N20	Thalamo-cortical radiations
P22	? Association projections
Peroneal	
LP	Dorsal roots and entry zone
P27	Thalamo-cortical projections
N35	? Association projections

Note: These origins are based on currently available evidence, and are not backed by extensive clinical-anatomical correlation. Therefore, these are subject to change.

Table 32.4 shows the postulated sites of origin of the waves comprising the median and peroneal SEP. Interpretation of abnormalities is as follows: A delayed EP with normal EP-N13 and N13-N20 intervals indicates a lesion in the somatosensory nerves at or distal to the brachial plexus. An increased EP-N13 interval with a normal N13-N20 interval suggests a lesion between Erb's point and the lower medulla. An increased N13-N20 interval with a normal EP-N13 interval indicates a lesion between the lower medulla and the cerebral hemispheres.

Some authors have interpreted N20 as coming from the thalamus, and P22 from the thalamocortical radiations. There is insufficient evidence to support such a conclusion. In practice, the important question answered by the median SEP is whether the lesion is in the periphery, spinal cord, or brain.

Amplitude abnormalities should be interpreted with caution. A marked asymmetry can be caused by a lesion affecting some but not all of the afferent fibers. However, if the lesion is not sufficiently severe to produce a latency change, then the study is probably normal. An absent N20 is abnormal when EP and N13 are present. If N13 is absent but EP and N20 are normal and the EP-N20 interval is normal, then the study indicates a lesion between the brachial plexus and medulla, but no statement can be made of brain conduction.

Ulnar Somatosensory Evoked Potential

For the ulnar SEP, the stimulating electrode is placed over the ulnar nerve in the lateral distal forearm, just before entry into the wrist. Recording electrodes, montages, machine settings, and analysis of results are identical to those described for the median nerve. Normal values should be established for individual laboratories.

Table 32.5 Peroneal Nerve Somatosensory Evoked Potential Stimulus and Recording Parameters

Number of trials	1,000-4,000
Stimulating electrodes	
Cathode	Lateral portion of popliteal fossa (PF)
Anode	3 cm distal to cathode
Recording electrodes	Spinous process of L3 (L3S)
	4 cm rostral to L3S
	Over T12 spinous process (T12S)
	4 cm rostral to T12S
	Over the T6 spinous process (T6S)
	4 cm rostral to T6S
	2 cm posterior to Cz (Cz')
	Midway between Fz and FPz (FPz')
Montage	
Channel 1	Cz'–Fpz'
Channel 2	T6S–4 cm rostral to T6S
Channel 3	T12S–4 cm rostral to T12S
Channel 4	L3S–4 cm rostral to L3S
Measurements	Distance from cathode to L3S
	Distances from Cz' to T6S, T12S, and L3S
	Peak latencies of L3S, T12S, and T6S potentials
	Peak latency of P27
Calculate	Conduction velocity from PF to L3
	Conduction velocity from L3, T12, and T6 to Cz'

Source: American Electroencephalographic Society 1986.

Peroneal Somatosensory Evoked Potential

Lower extremity SEPs are produced either by peroneal or tibial nerve stimulation. Selection depends on personal preference as well as on medical indication. Obviously, if a patient has a history of peroneal palsy and is undergoing SEP for evaluation of possible spinal-cord disease, the tibial nerve would be studied.

Peroneal Somatosensory Evoked Potential Stimulus and Recording Parameters

Peroneal SEP stimulus and recording parameters are shown in Table 32.5. The peroneal nerve is stimulated in the lateral popliteal fossa, just medial to the tendon of the biceps femoris. The cathode is placed proximally, and the anode distally. A ground is placed proximally on the same limb. The

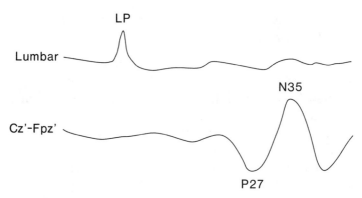

Figure 32.2 Peroneal nerve somatosensory evoked potentials. LP and P27 latencies are the only measurements routinely considered in interpretation.

stimulus intensity is such that each stimulus evokes a small twitch in the peroneal muscles.

The *Guidelines* recommends recording electrodes be placed as described in Table 32.5, as well as recording from multiple spinal levels as shown. However, the only measurements used for interpretation are latencies from L3S and the cortex (P27). The L3-P27 interval is sometimes called the *central conduction time.*

Peroneal Somatosensory Evoked Potential Waveform Identification

Sample peroneal SEP waveforms are shown in Figure 32.2. The reproducible waveforms with peroneal stimulation are a negative potential over the lumbar region, termed *lumbar potential* (LP), a positive wave over the cortex at approximately 27-ms latency (P27), and a negative wave over the cortex at approximately 35 ms (N35). A routine peroneal SEP study does not attempt to record from the cervical cord or medullary relay nuclei, since the amplitudes of these responses are very low when the leg is stimulated. Recordings from these areas require needle electrodes.

The waves are easy to identify. The LP is the most reproducible. The cortical potentials are best identified if at least two averaged traces are superimposed. P27 and N35 form a smooth waveform. The origin of the LP wave is the afferent volley in the lumbar nerves and cauda equina. The cortical potentials probably originate in the projections from the thalamus to the cortex. Some investigators have suggested that P27 is thalamocortical and that N35 is associative projections, but the clinico-anatomical evidence is not conclusive. Wave generation in this system is complex and it is difficult to attribute individual waves to specific locations.

Peroneal Somatosensory Evoked Potential Interpretation

The only important measurements are the LP and P27 latencies. A solitary abnormality of N35 latency and abnormalities of amplitude should not be interpreted as abnormal. Interpretation of the lower extremity SEPs is often made in conjunction with the upper extremity SEPs.

A prolonged LP with a normal LP-P27 interval indicates a peripheral lesion. The lesion may be in the cauda equina but is more likely in the peripheral nerve.

A normal LP latency and a prolonged LP-P27 interval indicates abnormal conduction between the cauda equina and the brain. Median SEP is required to localize the abnormality to the spinal cord. Normal median SEP indicates a lesion below the mid-cervical cord; prolonged median SEP indicates a lesion above the mid-cervical cord. However, a second lesion below the cervical cord cannot be excluded, since the P27 latency is already prolonged by the higher lesion.

A prolonged LP and an increased LP-P27 interval suggests two lesions affecting the peripheral nerve and central conduction. A single lesion in the cauda equina is also possible.

We have seen occasional patients with normal peroneal SEPs yet with prolongation of the central conduction with median stimulation. This is most likely due to the greater sensitivity of the median SEP to central disorders. If recordings had been made of cervico-medullary potentials from the peroneal stimulation, it is likely that the abnormalities would correspond to the median findings.

Tibial Somatosensory Evoked Potential

The tibial nerve supplies the gastrocnemius and soleus muscles in the leg, as well as the small muscles of the foot. While the sural nerve wraps around the lateral malleolus, the terminus of the tibial nerve wraps around the medial malleolus. In this location, the tibial nerve is superficial and can be stimulated for the SEP.

Tibial Somatosensory Evoked Potential Stimulus and Recording Parameters

Stimulus and recording settings are similar to those outlined for peroneal SEP. Specific recommendations are presented in Table 32.6. The proximal stimulus electrode (cathode) is placed at the ankle between the medial malleolus and the Achilles tendon. The anode is placed 3 cm distal to the cathode. A ground is placed proximal to the stimulus electrodes, usually on the calf. Stimulus intensity is set so that each stimulus produces a small amount of plantar flexion of the toes. Recording electrodes are placed as

Table 32.6   Tibial Nerve Somatosensory Evoked Potential Stimulus and Recording Parameters

Number of trials	1,000-4,000
Stimulating electrodes	Behind medial malleolus
Recording electrodes	Over tibial nerve in popliteal fossa (PF)
	Medial surface of knee
	Over L3 spinous process (L3S)
	4 cm rostral to L3S
	Over T12 spinous process
	4 cm rostral to T12S
	2 cm posterior to Cz (Cz')
	Midway between Fz and Fpz (Fpz')
Montage	
Channel 1	Cz'–Fpz'
Channel 2	T12S–4 cm rostral to T12S
Channel 3	L3S–4 cm rostal to L3S
Channel 4	PF–medial surface of knee
Measurements	Distance from ankle to PF
	Distance from ankle to L3 and T12
	Distances between spine electrodes and Cz'
	Peak latency of Pf potential
	Peak latencies of L3S and T12S spine potentials
	Peak latency of P37
Calculate	Conduction velocity between PF and L3
	Conduction velocities between spine and scalp

Note: Special circumstances may dictate changes in these standard parameters.

Source: Derived from American Electroencephalographic Society 1986.

shown in Table 32.6. Although the *Guidelines* recommended measuring potentials from T12S, measurements of these latencies are not normally used for routine SEP interpretation.

As with the peroneal SEPs, approximately 1,000 to 4,000 responses should be averaged, and at least two averages should be superimposed. Analysis time is routinely 60 to 80 ms; however, if the cerebral potentials are not identifiable, recording times of 100 ms or more should be used.

Tibial Somatosensory Evoked Potential Waveform Identification

The recorded waveforms with tibial stimulation include a potential recorded from the afferent nerve volley in the popliteal fossa (PF), potentials recorded over L3 and T12 spinous processes (L3S and T12S, respectively), and two potentials recorded over the cortex: P37 and N45. As

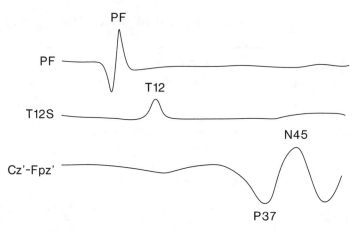

Figure 32.3 Tibial nerve somatosensory evoked potentials. Only PF and P37 are routinely used for interpretation.

with peroneal stimulation, recordings can be made from the cervical cord under special circumstances. A sample recording is shown in Figure 32.3.

Identification of the PF, L3S, and T12S waves is usually easy. Patients with peripheral neuropathy may have desynchronization of the afferent volley, such that the amplitude of the nerve potentials may be low or inconsistent. Interpretation of the cerebral potentials in this circumstance is discussed in the next section.

Identification of P37 and N45 is facilitated by overlapping averaged traces. The P37 and N45 form one smooth waveform that is followed by additional waves of no significance. P37 is the first reproducible positive wave recorded over the cortex. The P37 is identified by the prominent negative swing forming the N45.

Tibial Somatosensory Evoked Potential Interpretation

Interpretation of the tibial SEP is similar to interpretation of the peroneal SEP. The PF potential serves to monitor the stimulus and is of limited value if there are well-formed L3S and T12S potentials. If a peripheral lesion is contemplated, electromyography (EMG) with nerve-conduction velocity (NCV) would be done rather than making an interpretation on the basis of differences in PF-L3 interval.

A prolonged L3S with a normal L3S-P37 interval indicates a peripheral lesion. The lesion may be in the cauda equina but is more likely in the peripheral nerve.

A normal L3S latency and a prolonged L3S-P37 interval indicate abnormal conduction between the cauda equina and the brain. Median SEP is required to localize the abnormality to the spinal cord. Normal median SEP indicates a lesion below the mid-cervical cord; prolonged median SEP indicates a lesion above the mid-cervical cord. However, a second lesion below the cervical cord cannot be excluded, since the P37 latency is already prolonged by the higher lesion.

A prolonged L3S and an increased L3S-P37 interval suggests two lesions affecting the peripheral nerve and central conduction. A single lesion in the cauda equina is also possible.

Intraoperative Monitoring of Somatosensory Evoked Potential

Intraoperative monitoring of SEPs is performed chiefly for surgery on the spine, but recently has been used for cerebrovascular surgery. The waveform is not significantly altered by anesthetic agents. In fact, the waves are frequently much easier to record in an anesthetized, paralyzed patient.

Corrective surgery for scoliosis typically includes vertebral fusion and Harrington rod insertion. If there is no change in waveform or latency of the SEP, there should be no deterioration in neurologic function after the surgery. Clearly, this statement needs validation by careful study since, theoretically, there could be damage to the motor systems of the spinal cord, which are not tested with SEPs. A typical recording shows normal or prolonged waves of constant amplitude and latency through the surgery. The preoperative SEP may be abnormal because of compressive myelopathy from the scoliosis. If excessive stretch of the spinal cord occurs during insertion of the rods, there is either loss of amplitude or increase central conduction time of the SEP. Relieving tension on the spinal column results in the SEPs returning to the preoperative appearance.

Upper-extremity SEPs have been used during carotid endarterectomy to assess changes in the cerebral blood flow. If the cerebral waveform is lost, reduced in amplitude, or increased in latency, impaired conduction exists between the cervico-medullary junction and the cortex. One notable case from our own experience is an elderly woman who was undergoing endarterectomy for right carotid stenosis with an ulcerated plaque. Preoperative evaluation had found moderate atherosclerotic disease on the left as well. Throughout the surgery, the median SEP from the operated (right) side was stable; however, there was loss of the response from the unoperated (left) side. When the patient awoke, deficits from a left hemisphere infarction were evident. In this case, attention was focused predominantly on the operated side, but the loss of waves from the unoperated side correctly predicted subsequent deficit.

At Vanderbilt University Hospital, we stimulate the median or peroneal nerve continuously at a rate of 4.3/sec. Averages are continuously made, with

1,000 to 2,000 stimuli per average. The waveforms are continuously monitored by a technician, who prints a recording every five minutes. If there is any change in waveform or latency, the technician informs the surgeon, who considers the current procedure and may consult with the neurologist responsible for evoked potentials. The chief artifact during surgery is electrocautery, although there is potential for extensive artifact from the surrounding equipment. With artifact rejection and proper grounding, the effects of this interference are reduced to acceptable levels.

33

Motor Evoked Potentials

Motor evoked potentials are not routinely used by most neurophysiologists for several reasons. Special equipment is required, which is not expensive, but is usually not supplied with an evoked potential machine at time of purchase. Many physicians are afraid of liability associated with electrical stimulation of the brain, even though the risk of injury or kindling seizures is minuscule. Of course, there is a poor correlation between perceived medicolegal liability and the merit of the case. The biggest limitation to the use of motor evoked potentials is the clinical utility. New imaging techniques and sensory evoked potentials can provide most of the information that motor evoked potentials offer.

Physiological Basis

Motor evoked potentials are the responses of muscles to stimulation of the cerebral cortex and spinal cord. Since recordings are made only from the muscles, motor conduction velocities between cortex and spinal cord can be calculated. This is directly analogous to peripheral motor nerve-conduction velocities.

Delayed conduction of central motor axons can be produced by spinal-cord lesions, where there is compression or otherwise impaired action potential propagation. Structural lesions of the brain affecting descending motor axons and motoneuron degeneration can also produce abnormal motor conduction.

Methods

Stimulus

Electrical Stimulation

The method of stimulation can be electrical or magnetic, but magnetic is preferable. Electrical stimulation is anodal, as opposed to cathodal stimulation used for peripheral nerve stimulation. The most commonly employed technique uses a flat anode placed over the motor strip and a long belt-like cathode that goes around the head. Recording electrodes are placed over the muscle to be studied, which is often the abductor digiti minimi. The patient is asked to make a mild voluntary contraction of the muscle. This facilitates the response so that lower amplitude stimulation is required. Therefore, the field of anodal stimulation is very restricted. This prevents cortical stimulation from producing extensive muscle contraction.

The spinal cord can be stimulated near the C6 or T12 spinous processes. These are located to stimulate the cervical and lumbar enlargements, respectively. Voluntary activation does not facilitate the response to spinal-cord stimulation.

Magnetic Stimulation

Magnetic stimulation is provided by a hand-held coil of wire encased in plastic. Pulses of current are delivered through the wire. Charge movement through the coil creates a magnetic field like an inductor (see chapter 2, "Circuit Theory"). The magnetic field causes charge movement in cortical neurons. The cell bodies are depolarized and reach threshold.

Magnetic stimulation has several advantages over electrical stimulation:

1. Magnetic stimulation is not perceived as painful.
2. The skin does not have to be prepared as it does for electrical stimulation.
3. Neurophysiologists are not as concerned about the risks of magnetic stimulation as of electrical stimulation, even though the final electrophysiological result of both modalities is the same.

Recording

There are no universally agreed-upon guidelines for performing motor evoked potentials. The following were derived from King and Chiappa (1989).

Low-frequency filter is set to 3 Hz and high-frequency filter to 3,000 Hz. Gain is determined by the amplitude of the response. Set the gain so that the response produces a deflection that is at least 50% of the maximal excursion, but does not go off scale. Time base is set initially at 5 ms/div.

Recordings are made from arm and, occasionally, leg muscles. The following upper extremity muscles are most commonly examined: first dorsal interosseus, abductor digiti minimi, abductor pollicis brevis, biceps, and triceps. In the lower extremity, the tibialis anterior is most often studied. The active recording electrode is placed over the belly of the muscle. The reference is placed distally, over the tendon or distal joint.

Testing Protocol

Threshold Determination

The stimulus intensity is gradually increased until a compound motor action potential (CMAP) is seen. Then, the stimulus intensity is lowered to below threshold and successive stimuli given at regular incrementing intensities, for example 5% increase per stimulus. In this way, the threshold is clearly defined. For magnetic stimulation, the threshold is represented as a percent of the maximum output of the coil.

Motor Evoked Potential Recording

Cortical stimulation

The study is usually performed at rest and with facilitation. Stimulus intensity is set at 15% above threshold, and three stimuli delivered. The traces should superimpose. If they fail to superimpose, ensure that stimulating and recording electrodes are secure, and that the patient is completely relaxed.

Facilitation increases the size of the response while reducing latency. Many investigators believe a facilitated response to be more reproducible and therefore more clinically useful than a resting response. Facilitation is achieved by asking the patient to make a submaximal contraction of the muscle. The contraction should be about 10% of the maximal voluntary contraction of the muscle.

Spinal stimulation

Spinal stimuli are delivered at the level appropriate for the muscle being tested. For electrical stimulation, the stimulating cathode is just above or below the C7 spinous process. Best stimulation is obtained with the cathode in the space between spinous processes. For magnetic stimuli the muscles and levels are:

Biceps	C3
Triceps	C4
Abductor digiti minimi	C5

Voluntary contraction produces little facilitation of the spinal response, so it is not used.

Peripheral stimulation

The site of stimulation again depends on the muscle being studied. For biceps and triceps, magnetic stimuli are delivered to Erb's point. Electrical stimulation at Erb's point is much more painful and should not be used unless necessary. For hand muscles, electrical stimulation is delivered to the innervating nerves near the wrist.

Contraindications

Motor evoked potentials should probably not be performed in the following situations:

- Skull defect, such as a burr hole or craniotomy defect
- Metal in the head or neck
- Patient has a history of epilepsy or photoconvulsive discharge on EEG
- Patient less than 18 years of age.

Special caution should be employed in studying patients with metal or electronic devices elsewhere. Devices of special concern include pacemakers, implanted nerve stimulators, or implanted pumps (the magnetic field could conceivably change programming).

Interpretation

Measurements

Latency and amplitude are measured for each of the waves recorded using cortical, spinal, and peripheral stimulation. Latency is from the time of stimulus until the first deflection of the wave. Latency to peak of the response may be measured but is not used for interpretation. Amplitude is measured from baseline to the peak of the response.

Normal Data

Table 33.1 presents normal data for motor evoked potentials recorded from the abductor digiti minimi. Figure 33.1 shows a sample recording. Central motor conduction time (CMCT) is the difference between cortical la-

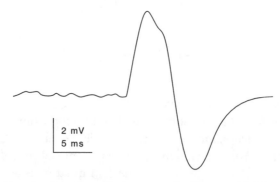

2 mV
5 ms

Figure 33.1 Sample recording of a motor evoked potential. Magnetic stimulation of the cortex and recording from the abductor digiti minimi.

Table 33.1 Motor Evoked Potential: Normal Data for Conduction

	Latency	*Amplitude*	*Interside Difference*
Cortical Stimulus			
At rest	23.8 ± 1.9	2.5 ± 1.3	11.1 ± 7.2
Facilitated	21.6 ± 2.4	6.9 ± 2.3	23.2 ± 17.1
Neck Stimulus	21.6 ± 2.4	7.1 ± 2.6	26.1 ± 27.4
Central Motor Conduction			
At rest	6.8 ± 0.9		
Facilitated	9.0 ± 0.7		

Source: Reprinted with permission from King and Chiappa. *Evoked Potentials in Clinical Medicine*, New York: Raven, 1989:520.

tency and spinal latency. Amplitudes are recorded but are so variable that they are not used extensively in interpretation.

Interpretation of Abnormal Responses

A response is abnormal if it is absent or if the CMCT is more than 2.5 to 3 standard deviations from the mean. Abnormalities may be seen from one or both sides. The CMCT is used for interpretation rather than absolute response latency, so that conduction in the peripheral pathways is not considered.

Increased CMCT is seen in a variety of disorders. Some of these are:

• Multiple sclerosis
• Spinal cord lesions
• Motor neuron disease
• Guillain-Barré syndrome
• Hereditary spastic paraparesis
• Stroke
• Coma

Multiple sclerosis (MS) causes prolonged CMCT in the majority of patients. Some patients may have only reduced amplitude. Suspected MS is probably the chief indication for motor evoked potentials, as an adjunct to visual evoked potential (VEP), somatosensory evoked potential (SEP), and magnetic resonance imaging (MRI).

Intraoperative monitoring is probably going to be the main use for motor evoked potentials. While SEP monitoring assesses the dorsal columns, supplied by the posterior spinal arteries, motor evoked potentials will assess conduction in tracts supplied by the anterior spinal artery. The two modalities will likely be used together.

Spinal-cord disorders frequently produce absence of the response or prolonged CMCT. Traumatic cervical myelopathy is almost always associated with abnormalities.

Motor neuron disease is characterized by absent responses. If present, the CMCT is only mildly prolonged. Some patients will have normal responses.

Pitfalls of Motor Evoked Potentials

Technical pitfalls are similar to those described for sensory conduction studies. However, there are some pitfalls specific to motor evoked potentials. Facilitation of the response to cortical stimulation requires that the patient make a voluntary contraction. Therefore, the muscle is active even prior to the stimulus. This can make determination of latency difficult. It can be hard to precisely localize the first deflection from baseline.

34 ⬜⬜⬜ ⬜⬜⬜ ⬜⬜⬜

Troubleshooting in Evoked Potentials

Noise

Most noise is due either to stray conductance or to stray capacitance. These electrical phenomena induce current to flow in electrode and amplifier wires, thereby obscuring the evoked potential (EP). Effects of stray capacitance and inductance are most pronounced if the electrode impedances are high or unequal. This is because unequal impedance destroys the noise-reducing benefits of the differential amplifier. See part I for further details on the mechanisms of noise and general principles on noise reduction.

Averaging of EPs can lead to errors in waveform identification. The most common averaging error is 60-cycle interference. If the stimulus frequency is a harmonic of 60 Hz, the 60 cycle can be averaged and obscure the recording.

Evoked potentials are typically very small in amplitude, but opportunities for noise interference are actually less than with most other neurodiagnostic techniques, due to the averaging required. Most sources of noise are not entrained to the stimulus, so that artifact and random noise are "averaged out." Potential error is possible if only one trial is performed. Even a single large-amplitude artifact can appear to be important after many averages. Therefore, superimposing at least two averaged trials is key to correct identification of the waves.

The stimulus rate must be selected carefully, so that 60-cycle interference is minimized. If the interstimulus interval is an even multiple of the interval between line waves (for 60 Hz = 1/60 = 16.66 ms) the line voltage may be very large in the amplified average. For a stimulus rate of 4.3/sec, the interval is 232.56 ms, definitely not an even multiple of 16.66 ms.

Even with artifact rejection and careful selection of stimulation frequency, EP waveforms are frequently superimposed on lower frequency waves. In this instance it is important to ensure that components of a sinusoid do not comprise a complex wave that could be confused with an EP.

Poor or Unusual Waveforms

Improper Electrode Position

As with most neurodiagnostic tests, the most common reason for poor results is poor technique. Improper electrode position will result in the wave being absent or in the wrong configuration. The most dangerous result is the misidentification of waves, leading to an error in final impression.

Improper electrode position is most common with the visual evoked potential (VEP) and somatosensory evoked potential (SEP). The landmarks for brainstem auditory evoked potential (BAEP) electrode position are more obvious. For the VEP, the electrodes may be placed either too high or too low on the occiput. If too low, there may be excessive artifact from muscle. Also, the amplitude of the waveform may be reduced. If the electrodes are too high, then the amplitude of the P100 may be reduced in amplitude or the waveform changed.

Anatomic Variability

Anatomic variation is a common reason for absent or unusual waveforms on evoked responses. The most common of these affects the VEP. Some patients have a tilt in the normal orientation of the dipole, making the region of maximum positivity more anterior than normal. This was described in detail in the section on VEP waveform identification, chapter 31.

Anatomic variation has very little effect on SEP and BAEP. In some patients, wave I of the BAEP cannot be identified. In this situation, it is important to use an electrode in the external auditory canal. This will aid in identification of wave I and distinction from the cochlear microphonic potential.

Polysomnography

35

□ □ □
□ □ □
□ □ □

Physiological Basis of Sleep and Sleep Disorders

Electroencephalography (EEG) during sleep was introduced in part II, "Electroencephalography." Sleep is used during routine EEG as an activation method to evoked epileptiform activity. Polysomnography (PSG) is the recording of EEG and other physiological parameter during sleep. The most common sleep disorders evaluated by PSG are narcolepsy and sleep apnea. Insomnia is probably the most common sleep disorder, but PSG is seldom of clinical value for this disorder. This section will cover the basic physiology of sleep and subsequently describe the methods and interpretation of PSG recordings.

Physiological Basis of Sleep

The sleep-wake cycle is controlled by the reticular activating system (RAS). The RAS consists of the brainstem reticular formation, posterior hypothalamus, and basal forebrain. These sites should be conceptualized as a continuous, though indistinct, structure rather than as separate nuclei.

The exact mechanisms of sleep and wake onset are not known. Activity in the pontine reticular formation, midbrain, and posterior hypothalamus are important for wakefulness. Activity in the medullary reticular formation is important for the generation of sleep. Sleep and wake may be integrated in the basal forebrain.

Wakefulness is probably a function of tonic activity in cells that project to the cortex. This activity increases neuronal excitability and may gate reactions to exogenous stimuli. Sleep develops as an active process that is generated by sleep-promoting neurons, such as the serotonergic raphé nuclei. This activation is probably promoted by a reduction in exogenous and endogenous stimuli that indicates a need for or an expectation of sleep. The tonic activating discharge and the response to exogenous stimuli are then suppressed, as are the patterned spontaneous activities normally seen while awake.

Years of sleep-deprivation experiments have not explained the need for sleep. The author believes in a computer model that sleep is required for data management. During the waking state, the brain receives a great deal of information on everything from music to tennis to physics. Much of this information is not ordered in a conceptual format; the brain cannot access the information in a structured way. For example, there is a great difference between owning a tape of a lecture and understanding its content. Some data processing can occur in the waking state, but sleep may be required to organize the day's input, integrate it with existing data, and perhaps discard seldom-accessed information.

Sleep Stages

Waking State

Electroencephalography in the waking stage was presented in chapter 12, "Normal Electroencephalography Patterns," and is summarized in Table 35.1. The adult waking EEG consists of predominantly fast frequencies. When the eyes are closed, a posterior dominant alpha rhythm predominates (Figure 35.1).

Stage 1

Stage 1 is usually separated into stages 1A (light drowsiness) and 1B (deep drowsiness). Stage 1A is characterized by desynchronization of the background, with loss of the posterior-dominant alpha rhythm. Theta activity is present but does not predominate (Figure 35.2).

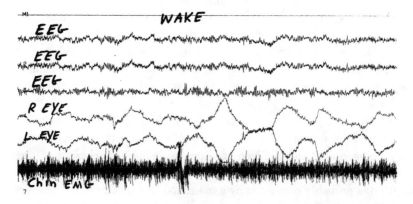

Figure 35.1 Waking state. There is a posterior predominant alpha with faster frequencies superimposed. Eye movements are conjugate.

Table 35.1   Sleep Stages

| State | Electroencephalogram | | | | | | | Electromyogram Activity |
	α	ß	θ	∂	V	K	S	
Awake	+	+	±	−	−	−	−	+
1A	±	−	+	±	−	−	−	±
1B	±	±	+	−	±	−	−	±
2	−	±	+	+	+	+	+	±
3	−	−	+	+	±	±	±	−
4	−	−	+	+	±	±	±	−
REM	−	+	+	+	−	−	−	−

For EEG: α = Posterior dominant alpha rhythm; ß = Beta; θ = Theta; ∂ = Delta; V = vertex waves; K = K complexes; S = Sleep spindles; + = Present; ± = May be present but not prominent; − = Not present to present to a minor degree.

For EMG activity: + = Present; ± = May be present but not prominent; − = Not present or present to a minor degree.

Stage 1B is similar to stage 1A except that slow waves, mainly in the theta range, appear. Vertex waves may be seen during this stage. Fusion of sleep spindles with vertex waves results in the K complex. Positive occipital sharp transients of sleep (POSTS) are seen during this stage.

Stage 2

Stage 2 is light sleep. The background consists of a mixture of frequencies (Figure 35.3). Delta activity is present although not as prominently as in deeper stages of sleep. Theta and faster frequencies are superimposed. Differentiation from Stage 1B is made by the appearance of sleep spindles. Vertex waves and K complexes are frequent.

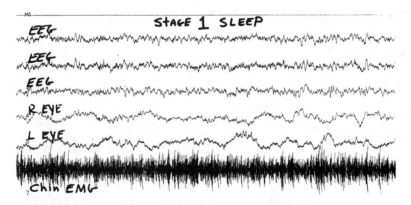

Figure 35.2   Stage 1 sleep. There is loss of the well-organized alpha, and the appearance of some theta.

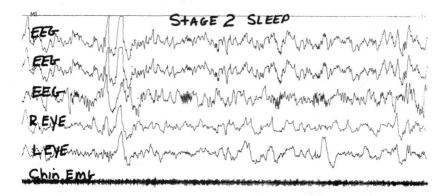

Figure 35.3   Stage 2 sleep. There are well-formed sleep spindles and vertex waves.

Stage 3

Stages 3 and 4 are slow-wave sleep. Stage 3 is characterized by delta activity with a frontal predominance. Sleep spindles, vertex waves, and K complexes persist but are not as prominent as during stage 2. Mittens are seen during this stage and are composed of a vertex wave fused to the end wave of a spindle. The small spindle wave is the thumb of the mitten and the slow vertex wave is the hand.

Stage 4

Stage 4 sleep is characterized by a predominance of slow activity in the delta range (Figure 35.4). The delta has a frontal predominance. While some faster frequencies may be superimposed, sleep spindles and vertex waves are seldom seen and, if present, are poorly formed.

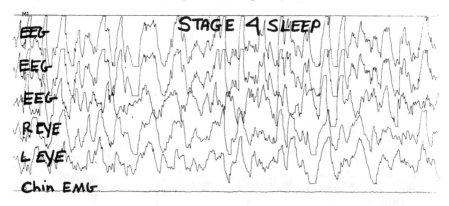

Figure 35.4   Stage 4 sleep. Delta activity predominates, with very little EMG activity.

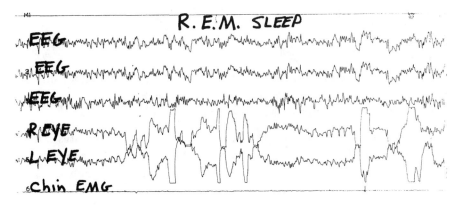

Figure 35.5 REM sleep. Eye movements are predominant, along with a mix frequency EEG pattern. There is little EMG activity.

Rapid Eye Movement Sleep

Rapid eye movement (REM) sleep is characterized by the predominance of low-voltage fast activity (Figure 35.5). Electro-oculography (EOG) and electromyography (EMG) recordings are especially helpful in differentiating this stage from a normal drowsy pattern.

Rapid eye movement sleep usually does not occur within sixty minutes from sleep onset. Sleep-onset REM is seen in patients with narcolepsy. Early onset REM may also be seen in some patients with sleep-deprivation, delirium tremens, and brainstem lesions.

Clinical Indications for Polysomnography

Polysomnography includes not only nocturnal sleep testing, but also multiple sleep latency testing (MSLT), and ambulatory PSG. Detailed indications for sleep testing recommended by the American Electroencephalographic Society, are presented below. Briefly, the following are general clinical recommendations that are open to personal bias.

1. Nocturnal PSG is indicated in patients who have clinical evidence for sleep apnea or who have excessive daytime sleepiness. These conditions suggest a nocturnal sleep disorder.
2. Multiple sleep latency testing is indicated when narcolepsy is suspected. MSLT can not be used to support the diagnosis of narcolepsy if the clinical history is not consistent. Excessive daytime sleepiness, alone, is probably not an indication for MSLT.

The *Guidelines'* official recommendations list the following indications for sleep monitoring:

- Episodes of sleep at inappropriate times
- Insomnia
- Hypersomnia
- Atypical behavioral events during sleep (for example, somnambulism, seizures, respiratory abnormalities, excessive movements)
- Assessment of effectiveness of treatment for sleep disorders.

Long-duration EEG monitoring of patients with suspected seizures usually does not require all of physiological monitoring commonly performed during PSG studies. However, measurement of some physiological parameters may be helpful, particularly in patients who may have autonomic components to the seizures.

36

□ □ □
□ □ □
□ □ □

Technical Aspects of Polysomnography

The technical recommendations for polysomnography (PSG) are taken largely from the *Guidelines for Polygraphic Assessment of Sleep-Related Disorders (Polysomnography)* 1991, published by the American Electroencephalographic Society. For the duration of this section, these recommendations will be referred to as the *PSG Guidelines*.

Polysomnography

Measured Physiological Parameters

The *PSG Guidelines* recommends that the following physiological parameters be measured:

- Electroencephalogram (EEG)
- Electro-oculogram (EOG)
- Submental electromyography (EMG)
- Electrocardiogram (EKG)
- Respiration
- Blood oxygenation
- Expired CO_2
- Body movement
- Behavioral observation
- Time

These parameters will be discussed individually. Not all laboratories record all of these parameters; however, this is recommended for accurate interpretation of the recordings.

Electroencephalogram

The *PSG Guidelines* recommends that at least six channels of EEG be recorded. The following electrode positions should be used as a minimum:

- Electroencephalogram (EEG)
- Electro-oculogram (EOG)
- Submental electromyography (EMG)
- Electrocardiogram (EKG)
- Respiration
- Blood oxygenation
- Expired CO_2
- Body movement
- Behavioral observation
- Time

These parameters will be discussed individually. Not all laboratories record all of these parameters; however, this is recommended for accurate interpretation of the recordings.

Electroencephalogram

The *PSG Guidelines* recommends that at least six channels of EEG be recorded. The following electrode positions should be used as a minimum:

- Fp1 and Fp2
- C3 and C4
- Fp1 and Fp2
- C3 and C4
- O1 and O2
- T3 and T4

Electrodes are attached using the same techniques described for routine EEG (chapter 10). Collodion is more dependable for long-term recording than the use of electrode gel alone, and is therefore preferable for PSG.

Montages are determined by the examiner, but should follow guidelines for routine EEG montages as described by the American Electroencephalographic Society (1986). Only one montage should be used to facilitate rapid sleep scoring. Paper speed for PSG is routinely set at 10 mm/sec, although faster speeds are occasionally helpful.

Electro-oculogram

Two channels are used for routine EOG recordings. Electrodes are placed in the following positions:

- 1 cm above and 1 cm lateral to the left eye
- 1 cm below and 1 cm lateral to the right eye
- Left ear/mastoid
- Right ear/mastoid

The two channels are each eye lead in reference to the ipsilateral ear. Using this montage, eye movements can be clearly differentiated from frontal slow activity. Eye movements will produce potentials of opposite polarity in the two eye leads. Frontal slow activity will produce either slow waves of the same polarity or independent slow waves in the two channels.

Submental Electromyogram

Submental EMG is recorded using standard cup electrodes placed underneath the chin. The electrodes are connected to a standard EEG amplifier with the low-frequency filter set at 10 Hz and the high-frequency filter set at 70 Hz. Gain is adjusted for each individual, but is in the same range as for EEG, about 7 μV/mm.

Submental EMG is reduced in deep stages of sleep and virtually abolished in rapid eye movement (REM) sleep. The absence of EMG activity aids in identification of REM sleep.

Electrocardiogram

The EKG is recorded using two electrodes on the chest, usually on the rostral sternum and lateral chest. Standard self-stick EKG electrodes are satisfactory. The low-frequency filter is set at 5 Hz and the high frequency filter at 70 Hz. Gain is adjusted for each individual but is usually set at approximately 75 μV/mm. Available settings differ between machines.

Recording of EKG serves two basic purposes. First, heart rate can change with respiratory distress, so that patients with sleep apnea and resultant hypercarbia and hypoxia may have initial tachycardia followed by profound bradycardia. In this situation, EKG gives an estimate of the severity of the apnea. The second purpose of EKG monitoring is to identify cardiac artifact in EEG channels. This is seldom a problem with PSG, because the technician should have minimized artifact prior to beginning the study. Also, bipolar montages greatly reduce EKG contamination.

Respiration

Diagnosis of sleep apnea requires knowledge of both respiratory effort and airflow. Respiratory effort is recorded using thoracic and abdominal strain gauge transducers, intercostal EMG, or thoracic and abdominal impedance. Airflow is usually monitored using thermal sensors near the nares and mouth. Alternating current (AC) recordings can be made if the time constant is sufficiently long (≥ 1 sec); however, direct current (DC) recordings are preferable.

Absence of airflow with preserved and even enhanced respiratory efforts indicates obstructive sleep apnea. Absence of airflow with depression in respiratory effort indicates central sleep apnea. Changes in respiration have to be correlated with blood oxygenation and expired air CO_2.

Blood Oxygenation

The pulse oximeter is most commonly used for measurement of O_2 saturation. Output of the oximeter is fed to the recorder by a DC-coupled amplifier, since absolute measurements require steady-state DC recordings. The oximeter is fastened to an earlobe or finger. The oximeter is fairly accurate, but may give a falsely high reading in patients with carbon monoxide in their blood (smokers). Oximeters may give falsely low results in patients with cool extremities or poor peripheral circulation.

Expired CO_2

Small tubes are placed below each nostril and near the mouth for sampling expired air. The air at end-expiration is largely alveolar, so that determination of CO_2 content is a fairly good indication of gas exchange. Patients with obstructive disorders will have a fall-off in expired CO_2 content during the obstruction, and may have higher CO_2 content after clearing of the obstruction.

Body Movement

A surface electrode is placed over the tibialis anterior on one side for recording EMG. This can reveal the presence of myoclonus and may aid in the diagnosis of restless legs syndrome. Alternatively, accelerometers can be used, which are small devices taped to the limb. Accelerometers produce a signal with a very small amount of movement. These are not used as much as surface EMG because of the expense of the accelerometers and the different type of connection to the input amplifiers. Submental EMG is already recorded, so placing additional EMG leads is conceptually and technically easier.

Behavioral Observation

Video monitoring of patient behavior using a closed circuit camera is essential. The other physiologic parameters can often be recorded by the same video tape recorder, after analog-to-digital conversion. Split-screen viewing of the video image, EEG, and physiological signals is desirable, although there is the potential for error if the resolution is not satisfactory.

The camera is positioned so that it can easily view the patient in bed. The camera should be able to provide a good image even in low light that is conducive to sleep. Additional light can be provided by infrared or ultraviolet sources. These light sources will activate the detectors in the cameras but will not alert the patients. Audio monitoring is provided by a sensitive microphone placed such that it can detect vocalizations and respiratory effort. The recording equipment should be located outside of the patient's room, so that machine noises and adjustments by the technician do not interfere with the patient's sleep. The most important aspects of behavior to observe are muscle twitches, signs of arousal, axial and limb movements, respiratory effort, and seizures.

Time

Time of onset and cessation of recording should be noted on the record. If a paper record is made, time can be calculated from the number of pages between onset time and an event. If a video recording is made, most video equipment provides for a digital time marker on the screen. Some laboratories record data on both videotape and paper. This is, in general, discouraged, because of the difficulty in precisely comparing events at identical times. Accurate time markers can minimize this error.

Recording Protocol for the Standard Nocturnal Study

The following guidelines summarize the requirements for a standard nocturnal study:

1. Make the room comfortable and quiet, with the recording equipment in a separate room.
2. Begin as close to normal sleep time as possible.
3. Minimize interruptions. Extra electrodes and sensors facilitate maintaining adequate recording if the patient dislodges primary electrodes and sensors.

Multiple Sleep Latency Test

The multiple sleep latency test (MSLT) is performed in the daytime and can be performed in standard EEG laboratories without special equipment. Patient preparation is minimal, although it is important to ensure that no sedatives are taken within one week of the test, since the results will be influenced by sedative drug effect or sedative withdrawal. The *PSG Guidelines* recommends performing the MSLT during the day following a nocturnal sleep study, so that the quality of sleep is known.

Conventional EEG electrodes are placed and a waking recording made. The patient is asked to go to sleep. The technician marks the time on the record.

The MSLT is performed as follows:

1. Patient has a normal night's sleep prior to the recording. Some neurophysiologists believe that it is important to have the patient under PSG study to evaluate the quality of the night's sleep. This helps to deter-

Table 36.1   Montages Used in Polysomnography

Electroencephalogram	C3-A2
	C4-A1
	O1-A2
	O2-A1
Electro-oculogram	OS-A1
	OD-A2
Electromyogram	Submentalis

Note: There are no official recommendations; however, these are adequate for staging routine records. Only EEG, EOG, and EMG channels are shown here. Other physiological parameters are measured as described in the text.

    mine whether a positive MSLT might be due to a disorder of nocturnal sleep, rather than be primary. A PSG recording is probably not necessary in all patients.

2. Electrodes are placed according to the 10-20 Electrode Placement System. The entire array is probably not necessary; however, it is easily placed in most EEG laboratories. If a limited array is placed, central and occipital leads are essential for identification of central vertex activity and the posterior dominant rhythm. (Samples of montages for EEG and noncerebral electrodes are shown in Table 36.1.) In addition to EEG leads, electrodes should be placed for monitoring the following physiological parameters:
   a. EOG
   b. Submental EMG
   c. EKG

3. At least four naps are begun at scheduled intervals. The technician lowers the lights and asks the patient to go to sleep. Approximately fifteen minutes of record are recorded before the first nap. After the "goodnight" command, recordings are made until the following criteria is fulfilled:
   a. Twenty minutes without sleep
   b. Fifteen minutes of continuous sleep
   c. Twenty minutes of interrupted sleep, even if less than fifteen minutes of sleep occurred.

37

Interpretation of Polysomnographic Recordings

Interpretation of Nocturnal Polysomnography

Sleep Staging and Interpretation of Nocturnal Polysomnography

Grading of sleep records is typically done in 20- to 40-second epochs. The 40-second epoch is convenient because this is the time for two pages of recordings at 15 mm/sec. An epoch is classified according to the predominant pattern during the epoch. For example, an epoch characterized mainly by a desynchronized background may be classified as stage 1 even though there is occasionally some posterior alpha activity.

Sleep onset is defined as either (1) the first of three contiguous epochs of stage 1 sleep, or (2) the first epoch of any stage 2, 3, or 4 sleep. Three consecutive epochs are not required.

With simultaneous monitoring of many physiologic variables, the amount of generated data can be overwhelming. The *PSG Guidelines* recommends the following sleep measurements:

- Total time in bed
- Duration of interspersed wakefulness
- Total sleep time
- Sleep latency
- Rapid eye movement latency
- Number of awakenings
- Time in each sleep stage (actual and percent).

Sleep efficiency is the percent of total time in bed spent asleep. In addition, graphs of sleep stage progression are drawn (Figure 37.1). These are usually done using simple computer programs.

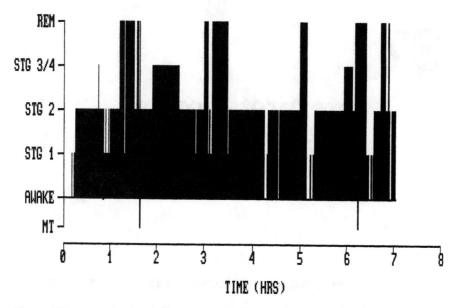

Figure 37.1 Histogram of sleep stages during a night of polysomnographic recording. This is a normal patient.

The following respiratory measurements are made:

- Rate in the wake and sleep states
- Presence of snoring
- Presence of paradoxical respiratory patterns
- Number and type of apneic episodes
- Frequency and degree of O_2 desaturation.

Electrocardiogram (EKG) data is analyzed for:

- Mean and range of heart rate during wake and sleep states
- Arrhythmias, if present
- Cardiac response to respiratory changes, for example, apnea.

Electromyogram (EMG) data is analyzed for myoclonus, and differentiation is made between myoclonus associated with arousal, myoclonus associated with epileptiform activity on electroencephalogram (EEG), and myoclonus not associated with other physiological changes.

Polysomnographic Findings in Common Sleep Disorders

Sleep disorders can be classified into the following categories:

- Hypersomnias
- Insomnias

Table 37.1 Polysomnographic Findings in Common Sleep Disorders

Narcolepsy	REM-onset sleep
Obstructive sleep apnea	Respiratory effort without air movement. Eventual arousal.
Central sleep apnea	Loss of respiratory effort during drowsiness or deep sleep. Eventual arousal.
Drug-related insomnia	Fragmented REM periods

Note: These are the most common distinguishing findings.

- Disorders of the sleep/wake cycle
- Arousal and paroxysmal disorders in sleep
- Excessive daytime sleepiness

Some investigators include seizures induced by sleep as a sleep disorder. However, this is really an underlying seizure disorder with sleep being used as an activating method. The neurophysiologic findings in specific sleep disorders are summarized in Table 37.1.

Narcolepsy

Narcolepsy is characterized by daytime sleep attacks. There are two types: (1) non-REM or isolated narcolepsy; and (2) REM or compound narcolepsy. Non-REM narcolepsy is characterized by non-REM sleep during attacks. Night sleep is normal. Patients with REM narcolepsy have REM sleep during their daytime attacks. At night, there is sleep fragmentation and shortened REM latency. The multiple sleep latency test (MSLT) may detect very short REM latency or sleep-onset REM. The MSLT tests naps, but may catch a narcoleptic sleep attack.

Sleep Apnea

Sleep apnea is probably the most common clinical reason for ordering polysomnography. There are three basic types:

- Obstructive or peripheral
- Nonobstructive or central
- Mixed.

All types are characterized by loss of air flow for ten seconds or more. Patients with obstructive sleep apnea continue to have respiratory effort that gradually increases because the movements are ineffectual (see Figure 37.2). Eventually, partial arousal results in opening of upper airway passages and restoration of ventilation. Patients with central sleep apnea lose air movement because of loss of respiratory drive. With subsequent hypoxia and hypercarbia, there is partial arousal and restoration of normal ventilatory effort.

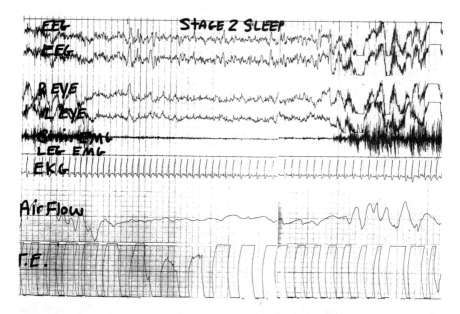

Figure 37.2 Obstructive sleep apnea. TE is thoracic effort or excursions. There is attenuation of airflow with continuation of thoracic effort. Eventually, arousal is accompanied by an increased effort, and movement of air.

Interpretation of the Multiple Sleep Latency Test

Measurements

The following physiological measurements are made: (1) latency from "goodnight" to sleep onset; and (2) latency from sleep onset to REM sleep. Forty-second epochs are scored according to the predominant background. If an epoch is mainly desynchronized with slow roving eye movements but does contain a small amount of posterior dominant alpha, the epoch is still scored as stage 1. Sleep onset is identified as the first of three consecutive stage 1 epochs, or any epoch of stage 2, 3, 4, or REM (Radke 1990).

Mean sleep latency is the average of the sleep latencies determined for each nap. Some neurophysiologists do not consider a test to be interpretable unless the patient falls asleep with two or three of the naps.

Interpretation

The most characteristic abnormality found on MSLT is short sleep latency. A mean sleep latency of less than five minutes is virtually diagnostic of hypersomnolence. Latency of ten minutes or greater is normal. A mean sleep latency between five and ten minutes is borderline. The report may indicate that consistent mean sleep latency of less than ten minutes is suggestive of a sleep disorder, but not diagnostic.

Mean sleep latency is altered by the following conditions:

- Sleep deprivation
- Certain medications, especially sedatives, antihistamines, and stimulants
- Withdrawal of some medications
- Age.

Withdrawal of medications such as benzodiazepines and barbiturates can have sustained effects; therefore, the medications should be stopped at least two weeks prior to the study.

Many patients with excessive daytime sleepiness will have shorter sleep latencies. Patients with narcolepsy will often have sleep-onset REM periods. The interpreter should be sure that the patient is not sleep-deprived before making the conclusion of sleep-onset or short-latency REM periods.

Glossary

Aliasing Alteration in waveform due to digital sampling at too slow a rate. Some frequencies may be mistaken for slower frequencies.

Alpha EEG activity in the 8- to 12-Hz range is alpha. This term usually is applied to the posterior activity seen in the waking state with the eyes closed (alpha rhythm), or the frontal activity seen in some patients with severe brain damage (alpha coma).

Alpha coma Coma due to severe brain damage, characterized by a relative loss of normal activity, and the presence of activity in the alpha range, most prominent in the frontal regions. This activity signifies a poor prognosis for functional recovery.

Ampere A unit of current. One coulomb of charge flowing past a point in a conductor each second is a current of one ampere (1 amp) (from Andrè Ampère, an eighteenth-century French physicist).

Amplifiers Magnify the signal so that it is large enough to drive a display unit. Ideally, it produces no change in the waveform of the signal.

Analog data Data is a continuous fluctuation in voltage. Compare with **Digital**.

Analog-to-digital (A/D) converter Electronic device that converts an analog signal into a digital signal using a defined sampling rate and voltage resolution.

Anode The positive terminal of a power supply.

Antidromic Stimulation of a nerve so that the action potential is conducted in the opposite direction to normal nerve impulse flow. Opposite of **Orthodromic.**

Axonotmesis In nerve trauma, breakage of the axons with the connective tissue sheath remaining intact.

Beta EEG activity above 12 Hz is in the beta range. Beta is most commonly seen in the frontal regions after sedation, and over surgical defects. This activity is normal.

Blink reflex EMG procedure. Brainstem reflex with stimulation of the trigeminal nerve and activation of facial muscles.

Breech rhythm EEG pattern characterized by a localized region of prominent beta activity. Usually due to a skull defect, giving less attenuation of cortical potentials.

Brief small-amplitude polyphasic motor unit potential   Descriptive term for myopathic motor unit.

BSAP or BSAPP   *See* **Brief small-amplitude polyphasic potential.**

Capacitor   A circuit element with the capacity to store energy in the form of an electric charge across two separated conducting plates.

Cathode   The negative terminal of a power supply.

Charge   A quantity of negatively charged electrons or positively charged holes. The unit of charge is the coulomb.

Circuit   A closed loop of circuit elements (such as resistors or capacitors) through which current flows.

Complex repetitive discharge   EMG pattern, usually considered abnormal. Repetitive discharge of several muscle fibers.

Conductor   A substance that is conducive to the flow of electrons. This type of material typically has unpaired electrons in orbitals that can fairly easily be encouraged to move within the material.

Coulomb   A unit of measure of charge. One coulomb is the charge carried by 6.24×1018 electrons (or holes) (from Charles de Coulomb, an eighteenth-century French physicist).

Current   The flow of charge. Can be described as either the flow of negatively charged electrons in one direction or the flow of positively charged holes in the opposite direction.

Decibel (dB)   A unit of measure of electrical signal intensity or sound intensity. For electrical signals, the number of decibels difference between two signals is equal to 20 times the log of the ratio of the amplitudes of the signals. For example, $1,000 \times$ difference = 60 dB.

Delta   Delta waves are EEG activity in the frequency range below 4 Hz. Delta waves may be single or multiple. Interpretation depends on the clinical situation. Delta activity is a normal component of sleep; however, delta in awake adult patients is always abnormal. The implications of delta activity differ depending on conformation and distribution. For comparison see **Frontal intermittent rhythmic delta activity** and **Polymorphic delta activity.**

Digital data   Data is represented by discrete data points over time. Compare with **Analog.**

Displays   Show the change in signal with time and location for meaningful analysis. Types include cathode x-ray tube (CRT) and chart (paper) display.

Dwell time   Sampling time of an analog-to-digital converter. This is the interval between samples. Preferred terms are **Sampling rate** or **Sampling interval.**

Early recruitment   Abnormal EMG pattern. With increased muscular effort, excessive numbers of units are recruited, because the contraction with each is inefficient.

Electron   A negatively charged atomic particle. It is the smallest unit of charge.

F wave   A motor nerve is stimulated and the response recorded from the muscle. The first potentials is the M response. At 30 to 55 ms, the secondary response is the F wave.

Fasciculation   Spontaneous discharge of a motor axon and its muscle fibers. May be normal, although it is seen in axonal neuropathies and especially motoneuron disease.

FIRDA.   *See* **Frontal intermittent rhythmic delta activity**.

Frontal intermittent rhythmic delta activity (FIRDA)   Abnormal EEG pattern. Episodic slow activity from the frontal regions, suggestive of a disconnection between deep nuclei and the cerebral cortex.

Frontal sharp transients   Spontaneous EEG sharp waves normal in neonates.

Fibrillation potentials   Spontaneous EMG activity. Due to single muscle fiber action potentials. Common in denervation and myopathies.

Filters   Simple electric circuits that deemphasize unwanted electrical signals. Common types are high-frequency filter, low-frequency filter, and 60-Hz filter. Filters may be active or passive.

14 and 6 positive spikes   Normal variant EEG pattern.

Grid   The signal inputs of amplifiers, for example, G1, G2. Derived from grids in tube devices.

Ground   A common reference for the patient and amplifiers. This may or may not be in continuity with the building ground.

H reflex   Electrophysiological equivalent of the tendon reflex, typically elicited by stimulation of the tibial nerve and recording from the soleus.

Hole   The "opposite" of an electron. More accurately represented as the absence of an electron. It therefore has a positive charge.

Impedance   "Resistance" of a circuit when dependent upon frequency. Used especially when a circuit involves capacitive elements.

Inductor   A circuit element that can store energy in a magnetic field created by moving charge.

Kirchoff's laws   Basic laws governing circuit theory (from Gustav Kirchoff, a nineteenth-century German physicist).

Lambda waves   Occipital waves thought to be related to visual exploration.

Leak current   The usually small amount of current that flows from a circuit through to ground. If a patient and equipment are not properly grounded, the leak current may be sufficient to affect electrically sensitive organs, such as the heart.

M response   A motor nerve is stimulated during nerve-conduction studies. The muscle is excited and the electrical activity recorded by surface electrodes. This is the M response.

Mu rhythm   Normal EEG rhythm. Central 10- to 12-Hz rhythm, characteristically abolished by movement of the contralateral hand.

Myopathic motor unit   Abnormal EMG pattern. Low-amplitude potential with multiple phases.

Myotonia   Repetitive muscle fiber action potentials, seen on EMG in myotonic dystrophy, myotonia congenita, paramyotonia congenita, and hyperkalemic periodic paralysis.

Neurapraxia   In nerve trauma, disruption of nerve fiber function without transection of the axons.

Neuropathic motor unit   Abnormal EMG pattern. High-amplitude, long-duration polyphasic motor unit potential.

Neurotmesis   In nerve trauma, complete transection of the nerve.

Noise   Loosely, recorded electrical activity that is unwanted for analysis. Strictly, electrical activity recorded that does not originate in the patient, but rather in the electrodes, wires, and/or equipment. This latter definition does not include muscle artifact.

Ohm   The unit of resistance. A 1-ohm resistance allows 1 amp of current to flow from a 1-V battery (from Georg Ohm, a nineteenth-century German physicist).

OIRDA.   *See* **Posterior intermittent rhythmic delta activity.**

Orthodromic   Stimulation of a nerve so that conduction of the action potential is in the same direction as normal nerve impulses is orthodromic. Opposite of **Antidromic.**

PIRDA.   *See* **Posterior intermittent rhythmic delta activity.**

Positive occipital sharp transients of sleep (POSTS) Normal EEG pattern. Occipital sharp waves seen in sleep.

Positive sharp wave   Abnormal EMG pattern. Muscle fiber action potential, seen in EMG recordings. Seen in denervating diseases and myopathies. Similar to fibrillation potentials.

Posterior intermittent rhythmic delta activity (PIRDA)   Abnormal EEG pattern. Similar to FIRDA, except with posterior predominance. Seen in children. Same implications as FIRDA.

Posterior slow waves of youth   Normal EEG pattern. Slow waves superimposed on the waking background.

Potential difference   The amount of energy required to separate a given quantity of charge. This is a measure of the ability to do work. This is measured in volts.

Power   Two meanings. (1) The rate at which energy can be transferred from a power supply to electrons. (2) The square of the amplitude of a specific frequency found after frequency analysis of a waveform.

Power supply   Imparts energy to electrons, which subsequently descend the electrical gradient toward the ground or opposite pole of the power supply. It may be a battery (DC), AC line power, or output of a transformer.

Pseudomyotonic discharge   Archaic term for complex repetitive discharge.

Reduced recruitment   Abnormal EMG pattern, characterized by a reduced number of motor units activated by voluntary contraction. Characteristic of denervating diseases.

Resistor   A circuit element that opposes the flow of electrons by dissipating voltage imparted to the electrons.

Sampling interval   Interval between samples measured by an analog-to-digital converter.

Sampling rate   Rate of sampling of an analog-to-digital converter. Sampling rate is the inverse of **Sampling interval.**

Secondary demyelination   Peripheral neuropathy due to damage primarily to the axon or neuron can result in some damage to the myelin. This secondary demyelination causes a slowing of nerve conductions, but to a much lesser extent than would be expected with primary demyelinating neuropathies.

Semiconductor   A material that is by nature a nonconductor but that has been doped with a material to slightly increase its conductivity.

Slow waves of youth.   *See* **Posterior slow waves of youth.**

Stimulators   Activate sensory nerve fibers to produce an evoked response from a biological system. Types include not only direct electrical stimulators but also visual and auditory stimulators.

Theta   Theta waves are EEG activity in the frequency band from 4 to 7 Hz. Theta activity is normal in young children in the waking state, and in sleep in patients of all ages. Theta activity in the waking state of adults is abnormal.

Time constant   For filters, the time taken for the response to a step change in signal voltage to return to 37% (1/e) of baseline. Measured in seconds.

Transducers   Transform biological energy into electrical energy. EEG and

EMG are already electrical and do not need transduction. Muscle tension and limb movements require transduction.

Transistor   A circuit element that uses one input to gate the flow through two other terminals. It is therefore a key element in amplifiers.

Volt   A measure of electrical potential difference between two points. This is the driving force for movement of electrons. One volt of potential difference can drive 1 coulomb of charge per second through a resistance of 1 ohm (from Count Alessandro Volta, a nineteenth-century Italian physicist).

Voltage resolution   A measure of the ability of an analog-to-digital converter to discern voltage differences. Determined by the number of bits of the converter. For example, a twelve-bit converter can define 4,096 (2^{12}) voltage levels. If the converter is set to have an analog input range of –10 V to +10 V, then the voltage resolution is 20/4096 = 0.0049 V.

Annotated Bibliography

American Electroencephalographic Society. *Guidelines in EEG and Evoked Potentials. J Clin Neurophysiol* 3, supp 1. (1986).

This is required reading for everyone who performs or interprets EEGs and evoked potentials.

American Electroencephalographic Society guidelines for polygraphic assessment of sleep-related disorders (polysomnography). *J Clin Neurophysiolo* 9 (1992);88–96.

Broughton, R. J. Polysomnography: Principles and applications in sleep and arousal disorders. In Niedermeyer and Lopes da Silva 1987.

Chiappa, K. H. *Evoked Potentials in Clinical Medicine.* New York: Raven, 1983.

This is an excellent review of the methods and interpretation of evoked potentials.

Chiappa, K. H. *Evoked Potentials in Clinical Medicine*, 2d ed. New York: Raven, 1989.

A comprehensive evoked potential text, covering all modalities described in this section, including motor evoked potentials. Required text for individuals who routinely perform evoked potential studies.

Cooper, R., and J. W. Osselton. Recording systems. In *EEG Technology.* London: Butterworths, 1980.

Most aspects of recording systems are discussed; particularly in-depth discussion of filters and the effects of the recording apparatus on frequency response.

Daly, D.D., and T.A. Pedley, eds. *Current Practice of Clinical Electroencephalography.* New York: Raven, 1990.

An excellent text. Complementary to Niedermeyer and Lopes da Silva 1987. Especially good figures. Accurate and easy to see.

Delagi, E. F., and A. Perotto. *Anatomic Guide for the Electromyographer.* Springfield, Ill.: Charles C Thomas, 1980.

Essential reference for neurophysiologists who perform EMG.

Delagi, E. F., A. Perotto, J. Iazetti, and D. Morrison. *Anatomic Guide for the Electromyographer. The Limbs.* Springfield, Ill.: Charles C Thomas, 1980.

Required reading and reference book for electromyographers. Excellent diagrams of needle positions for the muscles most commonly examined.

Dyck, P. J., P. K. Thomas, E. H. Lambert, and R. Bunge, eds. *Peripheral Neuropathy*. Philadelphia: W. B. Saunders, 1984.
In-depth two-volume text covering clinical, pathological, and laboratory features of peripheral nerve disorders.

Ekstedt J., Nilsson G., Stalberg E.; Calculations of the electromyographic jitter. *J Neurosurg Psychiatry* 37:526–39 (1974):291.

Hughes, J. R. Two forms of the 6/sec spike and wave complex. *EEG Clin Neurophysiol* 48 (1980): 535.

Kamp, A., and F. H. Lopes da Silva. Technological basis of EEG recording. In Niedermeyer and Lopes da Silva 1987.
Overview of basic electronics and electrical safety. Good discussion of strengths and limitations of EEG recording systems.

Kimura, J. *Electrodiagnosis in Diseases of Nerve and Muscle*. Philadelphia: F. A. Davis, 1983.
A comprehensive text covering most neuromuscular electrophysiological techniques.

Kimura, J. *Electrodiagnosis in Diseases of Nerve and Muscle: Principles and Practice*. Philadelphia: F. A. Davis, 1989.
A solid text for NCV and EMG. Not only covers the details of the individual tests, but also discusses some clinical aspects of neuromuscular disorders.

King, Philip S. L., and K. H. Chiappa. "Motor Evoked Potentials," In Chiappa 1989.

Kryger, M. H., T. Roth, and W. C. Dement. *Principles and Practice of Sleep Medicine*. Philadelphia: W. B. Saunders, 1989.
Comprehensive text on polysomnography. Considered the Bible by man sleep-disorder physiologists.

Liveson, J. A. *Peripheral Neurology: Case Studies in Electrodiagnosis*. Philadelphia: F. A. Davis, 1991.
Good annotated case presentations. This text discusses not only the implications of NCV and EMG findings, but also what studies are indicated, a subject not covered well by many texts.

Lombroso, C. T. Neonatal electroencephalography. In Niedermeyer and Lopes da Silva 1987.
Medical Consultants on the Diagnosis of Death to the President's Commission for the Study of Ethical Problems in Medicine and Biomedical and Behavioral Research. Guidelines for the determination of death. *JAMA* 246 (1981): 2184–86.

Miller, C. R., B. F. Westmoreland, and D. W. Klass. Subclinical rhythmic EEG discharge of adults (SREDA): Further observations. *Am J EEG Technol* 25 (1985): 217–24.

Misulis, K.E. Basic electronics for clinical neurophysiology. *J Clin Neuro-physiol* 6 (1989): 41–74.

Misulis, K. E., and G.M. Fenichel. Genetic forms of myasthenia gravis. *Pediatric Neurology* 5(1989):205–210.

Neidermeyer, E., and F. H. Lopes da Silva, eds. *Electroencephalography: Basic Principles, Clinical Applications, and Related Fields.* Baltimore: Urban and Schwarzenberg, 1987.

A comprehensive text of EEG. Most sections are well written. Basic electronics section contains a good discussion of strengths and limitations of EEG recording systems.

Polysomnography. *J Clin Neurophysiol* (1992).

Radke, R. A. Sleep disorders: Laboratory evaluation. In Daly and Pedley 1990.

Schaumburg, H. H., A. R. Berger, and P. K. Thomas. *Disorders of Peripheral Nerves.* Philadelphia: F. A. Davis, 1992.

Discusses the essentials of peripheral nerve diseases, including mononeuropathies. Not as comprehensive as Dyck et al. 1984, but very readable. All busy neurologists and neurophysiologists should read this book cover to cover and use Dyck's books as reference for specific cases.

Seaba, P. J., and D. D. Walker. Fundamentals of electronics and instrumentation. In Kimura 1983.

An excellent introduction to electronic instrumentation oriented primarily toward EMG. Much of the information is basic to EEG as well.

Sethi, R. K., and L. L. Thompson. *The Electromyographer's Handbook.* Boston: Little Brown, 1989.

Very practical book guiding especially nerve-conduction studies. Individuals new to NCV and EMG should have this book handy when learning the technique.

Index